PSYCHIATRY
CLERKSHIP

PSYCHIATRY CLERKSHIP

---

150 BIGGEST MISTAKES AND HOW TO AVOID THEM

Edited by Samir P. Desai, MD

Assistant Professor of Medicine, Baylor College of Medicine, Houston, TX

Authored by Kimberly D. McLaren, MD, Christopher D. Martin, MD, Paul Hebig, MD

PUBLISHED BY

MD2B

HOUSTON, TEXAS
www.md2b.net

The Psychiatry Clerkship: 150 Biggest Mistakes and How to Avoid Them is published by MD2B, P.O. Box 300988, Houston, Texas 77230-0988.
http://www.MD2B.net
Printed in the United States of America
ISBN # 0-9725561-5-X

Contents

Chapter 2 The Psychiatric Interview

Chapter 3 Prerounds

Chapter 4 On Call

Chapter 5 Write-Ups

Chapter 6 Presenting New Patients

Chapter 7 Daily Progress Notes

Chapter 8 Team Rounds

Chapter 9 The Oral Examination

Foreword

The clinical clerkship experiences of medical students may be likened to their taking a long trip (though hardly a vacation) through many different countries. The students are not "tourists" on these trips, but are immediately and intimately immersed in the vital life and commerce of the disparate nations that they are visiting. At the outset, the travelers are only vaguely familiar with the distinct languages, cultures and customs of the respective locales, and a significant amount of their time and efforts are expended in orienting themselves to such.

At about the time that the travelers have accommodated to their new environment and can begin to understand, learn from, and participate meaningfully in the community, they are suddenly transported to a different nation with new and unfamiliar language, culture, and expectations. Manifestly, the wise travelers prepare themselves for the journey by learning, *in advance,* as much as possible about the challenges that will face them when they first encounter their new destination. In that fashion their experiences and learning opportunities will be enriched by their not being distracted by having to learn the rudiments of communication and social expectation.

Although squarely rooted in the profession of medicine, the specialty of psychiatry is, perhaps, the most exotic of all medical specialties. There are several reasons for this. First and foremost, the brain is the most important and complex organ in the human body, and, arguably, the most important and complex functions of the central nervous system are cognition, mood and emotional regulation, perception, impulse control, and memory. These functions enable humans to think rationally and in abstractions, utilize language, and relate interpersonally and socially. These brain-based functions are responsible for human beings' superior capacities to adapt and survive. Manifestly, no organ in the human body works perfectly. When the brain fails to function adequately in the aforementioned realms, the diagnosis and treatment of patients affected thereby lies with province of psychiatry and neuropsychiatry. Because of the innate complexities and profound implications (for survival) of brain-based mental functions, dysfunctions therein are most difficult to understand and bear serious consequences.

I believe that far-reaching implications of brain-based dysfunctions of emotion, cognition and behavior are responsible for the historical stigmatization of the people who suffer from these conditions—and the mental health professionals who care for these people.

The manifestations of the stigmatization of the mentally ill are multifarious, and even encompass the people who, themselves, suffer from psychiatric disorders. Many people with serious psychiatric symptoms or disorders will not accept that they have these conditions and, therefore, refuse all help. This is quite different from most other medical conditions. Can you imagine someone who has a fracture of the patella or pelvis, or who is passing a renal stone, or who has acute pancreatitis refusing medical care? In addition, the very organ that is impaired must perceive that there is a problem and must be motivated to accept and capable of participating in the treatment thereof.

This unusual confluence of challenges explains, in part, why I consider psychiatry to be the most exotic and challenging of medical specialties. It also underlies why it is so difficult for—and important that--a medical student beginning his or her first psychiatric clerkship to "get the lay of the land."

Psychiatry Clerkship: 150 Biggest Mistakes and How to Avoid Them is a brilliantly-conceived and ingeniously-executed roadmap for medical students to approach and meet the many challenges of their psychiatry clerkship. As I read through this unique volume, I wondered why such an invaluable tool had not been crafted decades before.

The most common and deleterious mistakes that medical students might make during their clerkships are clearly presented, as are the best approaches to obviating such. Incidentally, almost all of these errors and the ways to prevent them have important applications to the practice of every clinical specialty. For example, I believe that it is no more salutatory to refer to a person as "a diabetic" than it is to label a patient as a "schizophrenic" or a "manic depressive." There is so much more to all of us than our ailments and dysfunctions.

Physicians failing to interact therapeutically with the family of a patient with cancer are no less neglectful than psychiatrists who ignore the parental input and involvement of a child with Attention Deficit Hyperactivity Disorder. It is just as important to ask a patient on an orthopedic service about alcohol and drug use as it is to do so on an inpatient psychiatry service. The accident that led to the fractured femur may have been caused by alcohol intoxication. I found the appendices in this text also to be jewels of advice and information about psychiatry clerkships.

The fortunate medical student who reads this text *before* the first day of his or her psychiatry rotation will be consummately prepared for what they are about to experience. Not only will this prepared medical student avoid painful pitfalls that are seemingly omnipresent on a psychiatry clerkship, but he or she will understand the rudiments of the specialty of psychiatry sufficiently to pay attention to and learn about the exciting subtleties of our field. For many medical students, their first exposure to the unique perspectives, knowledge base and skills of psychiatry is among the highpoints of their entire medical school experience. Vast unexplored vistas of understanding of themselves and others are opened up to them during their psychiatry clerkship. I wish the same for you and wish you the very best on your exciting and important journey upon which you are about to embark.

Stuart C. Yudofsky, M.D.
D.C. and Irene Ellwood Professor and Chairman
The Menninger Department of Psychiatry and Behavioral Sciences
Baylor College of Medicine
Houston, Texas

Preface

The psychiatry clerkship is often one of the most anxiously anticipated ones, even for students who have a number of other clerkships under their belts. A variety of factors contribute to this apprehension, including the need to learn a new psychiatric "language", to figure out how to interact with psychiatric patients, and the fact that the student must leave the comfort zone of the medical-style interview and examination. Once the initial anxiety is overcome, most students actually find the rotation very enjoyable.

The clinical experience is unlike any other, as it provides the luxury of spending more time with patients and getting to know them and their stories, as well as an opportunity to examine yourself and your reactions.

There are many books on the market focusing on the factual information you need to know for the psychiatry clerkship. While this information is certainly important for success on the clerkship, it doesn't actually prepare you for *doing* the rotation. These books fail to teach you how to approach patients, maintain your safety, and build rapport with patients. They don't prepare you for the usual daily activities of the rotation, such as rounding and writing notes. These are skills that each of us has had to develop, usually by making mistakes and having them corrected by our former residents and attendings.

In writing *Psychiatry Clerkship: 150 Biggest Mistakes and How to Avoid Them*, we thought of all of the mistakes that we made on our psychiatry clerkships and continue to see students make in our current roles as psychiatric residents and attending. In addition to pointing out these common mistakes, we offer advice on how to avoid making them yourself. We hope that you will be able to learn from our missteps and those of your predecessors and not be doomed to repeat them. By avoiding the errors made by most students (and perhaps by your fellow students who haven't read this book), you are certain to stand out on your rotation.

To secure the best possible evaluation on your psychiatry clerkship, we recommend that you review the first two chapters on approaching the psychiatric patient and conducting a psychiatric interview prior to beginning your rotation.

As you proceed through the rotation you can review the pertinent chapters to help you preround efficiently, compose thorough write-ups and daily progress notes, deliver polished and professional oral presentations, and impress the team during rounds. Additionally, if your institution uses an oral examination along with a written examination to evaluate students (a subject that is largely neglected in the current clerkship books), there is a chapter dedicated to helping you ace your oral examination. Finally, the reviews of psychiatric emergencies, major psychiatric illnesses and medications and other information contained in the appendices, will be invaluable resources to assist you in answering questions during rounds and preparing for your oral and written examinations.

Once you've mastered the concepts covered in this book, you'll be well on your way to success on your psychiatry clerkship. We hope you find your experience on your psychiatric rotation enjoyable, and we feel confident that this book will be a useful guide for your journey.

Kimberly D. McLaren, M.D.

Christopher D. Martin, M.D.

Paul R. Hebig, M.D.

About the Editor

Samir P. Desai, MD

Dr. Samir Desai serves on the faculty of the Baylor College of Medicine in the Department of Medicine. Dr. Desai has educated and mentored both medical students and residents, work for which he has received teaching awards. He is an author and editor, having written ten books that together have sold over 70,000 copies worldwide.

Dr. Desai is the author of the popular *101 Biggest Mistakes 3rd Year Medical Students Make and How To Avoid Them*, a book that has helped students reach their full potential during the third year of medical school. In the book, *The Residency Match: 101 Biggest Mistakes And How To Avoid Them*, Dr. Desai shows applicants how to avoid commonly made mistakes during the residency application process. He is also the editor of the Clerkship Mistakes Series, a series of books developed to help students perform at a high level during clinical clerkships and build the foundation needed for a successful career as a physician.

Dr. Desai conceived and authored the Clinician's Guide Series, a series of books dedicated to providing clinicians with practical approaches to commonly encountered problems. Now in its third edition, the initial book in this series, the *Clinician's Guide to Laboratory Medicine*, has become a popular book for third year medical students, residents, and physicians, providing a step-by-step approach to laboratory test interpretation. Other titles in this series include the *Clinician's Guide to Diagnosis* and *Clinician's Guide to Internal Medicine*.

In 2002, he founded www.md2b.net, a website committed to helping today's medical student become tomorrow's doctor. At the site, a variety of tools and resources are available to help students tackle the challenges of medical school.

After completing his residency training in Internal Medicine at Northwestern University in Chicago, Illinois, Dr. Desai had the opportunity of serving as chief medical resident. He received his MD degree from Wayne State University School of Medicine in Detroit, Michigan, graduating first in his class.

About the Authors

Kimberly D. McLaren, MD

Dr. Kimberly McLaren is a clinical instructor at the University of Washington in Seattle, where she supervises and teaches residents and medical students in the Harborview Medical Center Crisis Triage Unit. She completed her residency at the Baylor College of Medicine Menninger Department of Psychiatry in Houston, Texas in 2004.

During residency, Dr. McLaren received recognition for teaching medical students. She collaborated with other chief residents to organize a multi-disciplinary lecture series for residents in various specialty areas. She worked as part of a task force to develop a curriculum for a resident Clinician-Educator Track, one of only two in the nation that help prepare residents for careers in academia. She has also been active in organized medicine on a state and national level, and she has been an advocate for patients by lobbying lawmakers to shape legislative policy. She is the recipient of a 2004 American Medical Association Foundation Leadership Award and the American Psychiatric Association/Aventis Fellowship. Dr. McLaren plans to continue teaching residents and medical students with the goal of shaping the next generation of physicians. As a mentor, she hopes to encourage young physicians to take an active role in the future of medicine.

Christopher D. Martin, MD

Dr. Christopher Martin obtained his medical degree from Baylor College of Medicine in Houston, Texas, and was graduated in 2001. That year he entered his residency training in Psychiatry also at the Baylor College of Medicine. During the 2004-2005 academic year, he is serving as the chief resident of his training program, assuming clinical, educational, and administrative roles at The Methodist Hospital, the Michael E. DeBakey Veterans Affairs Medical Center, Ben Taub General Hospital, and other major teaching hospitals affiliated with Baylor College of Medicine. During his residency and chief year, he has helped to further the education of medical students, interns, and residents. Dr. Martin's career goals include practicing psychiatry as well as contributing to the advancement of psychiatric medicine and education.

Paul Hebig, MD

Dr. Paul Hebig grew up in New Hope, Minnesota. He acquired his bachelor's degree from the University of Florida in Microbiology. He completed medical school at the University of Florida in 2004 and has interests in addiction psychiatry and teaching. He is currently a first year resident at the University of Florida, in the Department of Psychiatry.

At the start of his medical career, he was interested in orthopedic surgery, but after he completed his psychiatry rotation during his third year of medical school and witnessed the drastic influence the appropriate psychiatric diagnosis and treatment could have on a patient's life, he knew that psychiatry was his calling.

ACKNOWLEDGMENTS

We would like to extend our grateful appreciation to all of our teachers and mentors, both past and present. We are fortunate beyond our ability to express gratitude that this list is too lengthy for inclusion here. We offer special thanks to Dr. Glen O. Gabbard, Dr. Joseph D. Hamilton, and Dr. Stuart C. Yudofsky for their contributions toward this work.

Chapter 1

Commonly Made Mistakes

Approaching the Psychiatric Patient

Many students begin their psychiatry clerkship with mixed anticipation because they are unsure about how to interact with psychiatric patients. While we cannot emphasize enough that persons with mental illness are just that, *people,* like you and me, you will need to consider the special needs that psychiatric patients may have. By better understanding how to approach patients on your psychiatry clerkship, you will be well on your way to having a fun and rewarding rotation. Mistakes commonly made by newcomers to psychiatry are reviewed in this chapter.

Mistake **#1**

Approaching the psychiatric patient like any other patient

While psychiatric patients and medical patients are more alike than different, your approach should be tailored to the specific needs of the patient. Evaluating a psychiatric patient will require you to listen more and talk less. You will need to listen not only to what your patients are saying, but also to how they are saying it, what their body language is saying, and what they are not saying. All of these factors are imperative in successfully evaluating patients on your psychiatry clerkship.

1

Mistake **#2**

Regarding the patient as a disease

Although psychiatric patients suffer from disease states that may intimately influence their emotions and expression of personality, we must not fall into the trap of forgetting that there is always a person with genuine emotions and an authentic personality underneath the illness itself. This mistake is best avoided by remembering that a patient who has schizophrenia is a person with schizophrenia, not a schizophrenic. It follows that a patient must also always be referred to as such: a person, not a disease. This concept should be applied to all patients, not just those you encounter on your psychiatry rotation.

Success Tip #1

Don't refer to a patient as a disease. This will help you remember that though they have an illness, they are people first and foremost.

Mistake **#3**

Looking in your pocket for tools to evaluate and treat psychiatric patients

Unlike other rotations in which you have pockets full of diagnostic tools and examination equipment, your most important tool for your psychiatry rotation will be yourself. You will need to listen attentively, not only to the patient, but also to your own feelings about the patient. For instance, the patient reporting a severe depression should invoke feelings of sadness in you. If you are not experiencing any feelings, you may not be empathically tuned in to the patient or the patient may not truly be depressed. Your gut reaction to patients will help you determine how ill they are and what treatment is necessary.

Success Tip #2

Use this rotation to develop your gut instinct. Ask your attending how the patient makes them feel as a reference. You will find that you can actually become more in tune with this instinct if you practice. This will serve you well no matter what field of medicine you decide on, as well as in the world outside of medicine.

Mistake #4

Not keeping your reactions to patients in check

One of the most interesting things about psychiatry is hearing all sorts of stories from patients. These stories are often disturbing, bizarre, and at times, even comical. However, it is important that your emotional response to these stories not become an obstacle to the patient's disclosure. Especially in the case of a psychotic patient, you will need to put on your "poker face" in order to encourage the patient to elaborate on his delusions, which may seem completely outlandish to you. If you do not keep your reactions in check and the patient feels that you do not understand him or her, you will not be able to treat that patient effectively.

Mistake **#5**

Dressing inappropriately

As is the case with your other rotations, you should always dress neatly. Many psychiatrists wear a white coat in the hospital, but may not in an outpatient clinic. Scrubs may be appropriate when you are on call or in an emergency center setting, but otherwise professional dress will be expected. You should look to your attending or resident to determine what is most appropriate. If you are working in a psychiatry emergency center or on an inpatient unit with patients who are severely ill, you should not wear neckties or long jewelry that could be grabbed by an agitated patient. You may also want to avoid clothing or shoes that would make it difficult to make a quick escape if necessary.

Success Tip #3

Pattern your dress after your resident or intern, who will have similar interactions with patients. Don't wear anything that could be used as a weapon by an agitated patient (i.e., neckties or long, dangling jewelry).

Mistake **#6**

Neglecting your personal safety

Though most patients will not pose a danger to you, some patients, especially those who are paranoid or intoxicated, may become violent. When evaluating and working with psychiatric patients, whether in an emergency center, inpatient unit, or outpatient clinic, it is important to keep one's personal safety in mind. Several rules apply here. The environment in which interactions with patients occur should be controlled. Objects that might be thrown or otherwise used as weapons should not be within the patient's reach. The interviewer should sit closest to the door of the room, which may be left open so that a prompt exit may be made if the patient becomes agitated. The placement of a desk between the interviewer and patient may also aid in such instances. It is also important to listen to your "gut." If you are feeling uneasy or frightened, you should immediately end the interview.

Mistake #7

Failure to pay attention to cues from the patient

In addition to listening to your own inner cues that a situation is becoming dangerous, you also need to pay attention to the patient. Even a patient who is very psychotic can often let you know when he has had enough. It is important to observe the patient for escalating psychomotor agitation, increased movements of the arms and legs, clenching of fists, pounding on walls or desks, etc. Verbal threats should also be taken seriously and are grounds for immediate termination of an interview. Should a patient become physically agitated or threatening, one should try to de-escalate the situation, using verbal interventions to reassure the patient in soft, calm tones and non-threatening hand gestures. If you feel threatened, leave the room quickly and calmly.

Success Tip #4

Practice listening to your "gut" reaction when interviewing psychiatric patients. Also, pay attention to how the patient is tolerating the interview. If you feel threatened by a patient, end the interview. Safety—the patient's as well as yours—outweighs the importance of information gathering.

Mistake **#8**

Thinking of yourself as the lone ranger

Most emergency room and inpatient settings have staff members who are specially trained in dealing with psychiatric patients. These staff members are invaluable in helping you take care of patients. They often know the patients better than you or the resident and can let you know if the patient has a tendency to become violent. They may also accompany you while you interview patients until you feel comfortable. Chapter 8 contains more information about the members of the treatment team and the roles they play.

Mistake **#9**

Assuming that all psychiatric patients are dangerous

While we have just reviewed how to protect yourself while interacting with psychiatric patients, it is important to point out that the vast majority of patients that you will see on your psychiatry clerkship will not pose a threat to

6

your personal safety. Discomfort with mental illness often leads to fear of psychiatric patients. Additionally, media portrayals of mental illness have exacerbated this dynamic, encouraging the belief that persons suffering from mental illness are typically violent criminals or psychopathic madmen. In reality, psychiatric patients are seldom threatening, and when understood and approached appropriately, they are even less likely to be dangerous. When interacting with a patient it is important not to let fear interfere with your ability to appreciate, understand, and care for the human being. To do so would prevent you from functioning as an effective physician.

Mistake #10

Neglecting the role of the patient's family

In psychiatry more than any other field, except perhaps pediatrics, it is essential to include the family, if available, in the evaluation and treatment of the patient. Patients with severe and disabling mental illness may not be able to provide an accurate history of their premorbid functioning, symptoms, and course of treatment. All of this information is vital to the evaluation and continued care of the patient. Therefore, it is of great importance to communicate with the family in the early stages of evaluation and treatment of the patient. Because you may have more contact with the family than any other member of the treatment team, they may also look to you to answer their questions about what is going on with their loved one. It is never appropriate for you to give information that you are unsure of. Rather, let the family know that you appreciate their concerns, will discuss them with the team, and will get back to them.

Remember that talking with family generally requires your patient's consent. Mistake #15 discusses confidentiality in more depth.

Mistake *#11*

Not appreciating the patient's baseline functioning

Patients with chronic mental illness such as schizophrenia, bipolar disorder, or recurring severe major depressive disorder will experience an exacerbation of their conditions at times. They may thus require acute hospitalization when their illness threatens their own safety or the safety of others. When this type of patient is evaluated in the hospital, the goal is to return them to the best functional level possible given their chronic condition. For this reason, it is important to understand how well the patient functions when stabilized to the best of current medical ability. Reviewing the chart and talking with family and friends can help determine the patient's baseline functioning.

Success Tip #5

Collateral information from the patient's family or friends can help in determining the baseline functioning. The goal of treatment is to return the patient to this level of functioning (or better if possible).

Mistake #12

Not regarding mental illnesses as medical illnesses

Those who are unfamiliar with the field of mental health may at first fail to understand that mental illnesses are truly medical illnesses that cause significant distress and functional impairment. One myth our culture has created is that of the eccentric madman, an unusual character possessing a unique personality and special wisdom who is treated against his will by the mental health system so he will conform and become "normal." While certainly each individual does possess unique and valuable personal attributes, those individuals who meet criteria for a psychiatric disorder such as schizophrenia, bipolar disorder, or major depressive disorder have a brain disease. Their neuro-circuitry is not functioning normally. There is irrefutable evidence that these patients have *physiologic* problems. Understanding mental illness as medical illness will help you approach patients in a more empathic way.

Mistake #13

Overlooking the contribution of underlying medical illness

Of course, the distinction here becomes rhetorically awkward because we know that all psychiatric illness is physiologically based medical illness. However, when working in psychiatry it is important not to make the mistake of only thinking of primary psychiatric disorders when evaluating a patient and generating a differential diagnosis. Many general medical conditions may masquerade as primary psychiatric illness. For instance, thyroid disease, myocardial infarction, neurological disease and intracranial neoplasms, among others, may all present initially with psychiatric symptoms. It is important to maintain a degree of suspicion for general medical conditions when evaluating patients so that medical disease and its appropriate treatment are not overlooked.

Mistake #14

Overlooking the contribution of psychoactive substance use

Similarly, intoxication and withdrawal from a number of psychoactive drugs may lead to psychiatric symptoms. This includes drugs of abuse, as well as medications prescribed appropriately by physicians, such as corticosteroids, interferon, beta blockers and benzodiazepines, just to name a few. So, clearly, when evaluating patients it is crucial to obtain a history of all medications the patient is taking. Also, with each patient seen in psychiatry it is crucial to develop a thorough history of their past and present use of alcohol and illicit drugs.

Success Tip #6
General medical illness and psychoactive substance use and/or withdrawal can produce psychiatric symptoms and mimic psychiatric illness. Don't overlook non-psychiatric etiologies of presenting symptoms. To do so may be lethal for the patient!

Mistake **#15**

Breaching patient confidentiality

Though there are now federal regulations in place to protect the confidentiality of all patients' health care information, it is of the utmost importance to protect psychiatric patients' privacy. No other medical information, with the possible exception of genetic data, can be used to discriminate against a patient like information about their mental health. For this reason, we go to great lengths to protect the privacy of psychiatric patients. You are not allowed to disclose whether a patient is under the care of a psychiatrist or whether they are or have been hospitalized for psychiatric reasons without the patient's explicitly stated permission. You should ask the patient for permission to give and/or receive information. With sensitive information, be sure to ask the patient specifically if that information can be shared.

The exception to this rule is an emergency situation. For example, if a patient presents to the emergency department and is unable to give any coherent historical information about himself, you may contact family, if known, for more information. Even in a case like this, it is generally better to listen to information presented by family and limit the information that you give them. As always, you should not talk about patients in public places or give patient information to anyone that is not a part of the treatment team.

Success Tip #7

Maintaining confidentiality is of paramount importance in psychiatry. Always ask the patient and document in the medical record their consent for you to speak with anyone else about them and their illness.

Chapter 2

Commonly Made Mistakes During

The Psychiatric Interview

During other clerkships you may rely on physical examination and diagnostic procedures to help in making diagnoses. While on your psychiatry clerkship, however, your primary diagnostic tool will be your psychiatric interview. The way in which you interact with patients and perform the interview will likely comprise a large component of your grade. This chapter reviews common mistakes made while conducting a psychiatric interview.

Mistake **#16**

Doing most of the talking

As alluded to in the last chapter, interviewing psychiatric patients involves more listening than talking. You should begin with open-ended questions like "What brings you here today?" or "What can we do for you?" that allow the patient to express his or her primary reasons for seeing you. You can then narrow your questions to get more specific information. If you begin with closed-ended questions and interrupt the patient repeatedly, you will get very limited information, and the patient will not feel that his or her needs have been adequately addressed.

Mistake **#17**

Not being tuned in to the patient

You will hear about the concept of empathy from the first day of your psychiatry rotation. Empathy can be defined as the capacity to understand and vicariously share in the feelings, thoughts, and experiences of another without that person having to explicitly state what they are. This is a skill that some people have naturally, and most everyone can develop. The initial interview begins the process of establishing rapport with the patient and sets the tone for all interactions and treatment interventions to follow. Therefore, it is important that the patient feels that the two of you have established an empathic connection early on. The patient will feel appreciated and understood and that you are listening to his concerns. A great psychiatrist said of being with patients, "When in doubt, be human." Having an empathic connection with your patients will help you to treat them as human beings.

Success Tip #8
When in doubt, be human.

Mistake **#18**

Using a scripted interview format

Though there are certain questions that you must ask every patient (these will be discussed later in this chapter), it is important that your interview be a dance in which you often let the patient lead. Let your patient do a significant portion of the talking and be empathic, as discussed above. It also means that you give the patient some latitude in choosing what he or she wants or needs to talk about. Allowing the patient to take the lead at times in the interview will ultimately make it a more productive and informative interview, as well as establish an important rapport. The interview should be more like a *conversation* than a *list of questions.* It would be an empathic failure to follow the patient's emotional revelation of a history of childhood abuse with a question such as, "How is your sleep?" A good rule of thumb is to speak with the patient as if you were having a conversation, and remember always to be human.

You will probably want to take some notes during your conversational interview, and it may be helpful to let the patient know that you will be doing so at the beginning of the interview. Don't let your note-taking interfere with your conversation. Practice taking notes while maintaining eye contact with the patient.

Mistake **#19**

Failure to focus the interview sufficiently

While it is important to initiate interviews in an open-ended fashion and to follow the patient's lead at times, it is also essential that the interview then focus on gathering the information that will allow for the formulation of a diagnosis and the initiation of treatment within an appropriate period of time. One method that will assist with this goal is to structure the body of the interview along the major categories of psychiatric illness. Use screening questions to focus in an organized fashion on mood, anxiety, psychotic, and substance abuse symptoms. You can then move on to other important areas of the assessment that will be discussed later in this chapter. You may need to interrupt and redirect the patient in order to accomplish all that is necessary in a given time. You may say, for example, "I would like to hear more about your difficulties at work, but we need to move on so that we can cover everything before we run out of time." This approach conveys to the patient that you are interested in what they are saying but also want to learn everything necessary to treat them appropriately.

Success Tip #9

Begin with open-ended questions and then narrow your focus to get more specific information. The interview should flow like a conversation, rather than a list of questions.

Mistake **#20**

Not making the patient feel comfortable

Especially when interviewing a patient during team rounds, it is important to make the patient feel comfortable. This can begin with allowing the patient to choose his seat and position it a comfortable distance from the interviewer. You should then have members of the team introduce themselves and state their role in the treatment. It also helps to explain to the patient that the purpose of the team interview is so that all of the people who need to get to know the patient can do so at the same time, reducing the redundancy of multiple interviews. Part of being empathic is noting when a patient is feeling uncomfortable. A statement such as "It must be difficult to answer all of these questions in front of so many people, and we appreciate your courage in doing so" can go a long way toward putting the patient at ease. As you ask more pointed questions, note the patient's ability to deal with the anxiety and painful affects which may be generated and comment on this to the patient. You can use this as an opportunity to make an empathic connection with the patient.

Mistake #21

Making assumptions about the patient's meaning

You should not assume that you know what patients mean when they tell you about their feelings or experiences. For instance, a patient may tell you that their father was mean and abusive. For a sensitive patient, this may mean that her father never hugged her or told her that he loved her. For another patient, this may mean that his father yelled insults and beat him every day. It is always important to ask the patient to elaborate and to clarify your understanding of what has been said. This technique will not only insure that you get an accurate history, but will also give you clues about how the patient may experience you.

Success Tip #10
Clarifying what the patient says will result in a more accurate history, and the patient will feel better understood by you.

Mistake **#22**

Disclosing personal information

While the initial interview is not the only time that one could disclose personal information to a patient, it is an important point to make here. In psychiatry, more so than in any other medical specialty, there are very specific and stringent professional guidelines with respect to certain behavior with patients. There is an intimacy that exists between the patient and mental health professional that places the patient in a very vulnerable position. It should go without saying that you must avoid any sexual activity with patients. Similarly, any behavior that may be a prelude to sexual activity or other boundary violations should be avoided. This includes disclosing personal information to the patient. While some of the things that patients tell you may resonate with your own personal experience, which can help you feel more empathic toward a patient, it is generally not appropriate to share this information with the patient. To do so may cause a shift in the dynamics of the relationship, which could potentially be harmful to the patient. For instance, if a patient is having problems in a relationship, you might be tempted to say that you are also having a difficult time with your significant other. While this could be seen as letting the patient know that you understand what they are going through, it would also put the patient in a position of having to worry about and take care of you, rather than the other way around.

There is wide variation in what may be appropriate to disclose to various types of patients. Generally, a psychiatrist may disclose more about themselves to those patients who are more severely ill, elderly, or lower functioning than to higher functioning patients in psychotherapy. A good rule of thumb is to think about why you want to disclose personal information to a patient. Is it to help the patient or to help yourself? When in doubt, ask your resident or attending before self-disclosing.

Mistake **#23**

Appearing judgmental

In psychiatry, it is of particular importance that patients feel free to speak about whatever is on their mind, without fear of being judged. Patients may have problems of which they are embarrassed or ashamed, yet they need to feel free to discuss these matters with you, their caregiver. Also, when on your psychiatric rotation, as well as when rotating through other specialties, you will encounter patients with diverse backgrounds and lifestyles, often different from your own. If patients sense that you are uncomfortable with them or seem to judge them, they will be unable to trust you with information that may be vital to their evaluation and treatment. It is of the utmost importance when interviewing, and at all other times as well, that you present yourself to all patients in a nonjudgmental, supportive, and caring manner so that they may feel comfortable sharing sensitive information with you.

Mistake **#24**

Neglecting to inquire about suicide

There are a number of things about which you must inquire with every patient, or you will fail your rotation. The most important of these is suicidality. The proper evaluation of the suicidal patient will be one of the most useful things that you will learn on the psychiatry clerkship. Patients with severe psychiatric illness such as major depression, bipolar disorder, and schizophrenia, to name a few, are at significant risk of committing suicide. For this reason, it is important that your evaluation of every patient include an assessment of suicide risk. It is best that this be done directly. You may start by asking an open-ended question such as, "Have things gotten so bad that you have thought life is not worth living?" If the patient answers in the affirmative, you should proceed to ask more specific questions such as, "Have you thought about taking your own life?" and "Have you thought of a specific plan for how you might accomplish this?" There is a myth that asking depressed patients about suicide will somehow plant this idea in their mind. It is far more likely that a depressed patient has already thought of suicide long before you ask them about it. It is highly unlikely that your inquiring about suicide will make patients any more likely to attempt to take their life. In fact, not asking about suicide is far worse, and may constitute malpractice.

Success Tip #11
You must ask every patient about suicidal ideations.

Success Tip #12
Asking a patient about suicidality will not plant the idea in his mind.

Mistake **#25**

Failure to ask about substance abuse

There is a high rate of co-morbidity between psychiatric illness and the abuse of alcohol and drugs. Many individuals suffering from psychiatric illness will turn to alcohol and drugs of abuse in an attempt to self-medicate their suffering. Also, the abuse of alcohol and other drugs will often lead to the development of psychiatric symptoms including anxiety, mood disturbances, and psychosis. Therefore, whenever interviewing in a psychiatric setting, it is essential that *every* patient be asked about the use of alcohol and other substances. Here again, the direct approach is best. A patient may be asked, "How much do you drink?" and "Do you use any other drugs like marijuana, cocaine, uppers, or downers?" Prescription drug abuse may be addressed with, "Do you take any medications other than those prescribed by your doctors?" Asking these questions in a direct and nonjudgmental way increases the likelihood that you will get an honest answer. Also, be sure to ask about history of blackouts, withdrawal symptoms, seizures, delirium tremens, and prior detox treatments.

Success Tip #13
Every patient should be asked directly about alcohol and drug use.

Mistake #26

Forgetting to inquire about family history

Psychiatric illness is heavily genetically influenced. Often, a patient's family history may be very enlightening when working to formulate a diagnostic picture. A history of mental illness in the family may support a given diagnosis in your patient. A family history of suicide may increase the patient's risk of dying by suicide as well. Also, a history of response to a given medication in a first-degree relative may indicate that your patient is likely to respond well to the same medication. These pieces of information are all potentially useful and easily obtained by asking about the patient's family history.

Mistake #27

Failure to ask about medical history

As discussed in the last chapter, many medical conditions may mimic psychiatric illness. It is important to ask the patient about his medical history and to maintain a level of suspicion of medical illness.

Mistake #28

Neglecting the significance of the psychosocial history

In psychiatry it is crucial to gain an understanding of the patient's social situation. The environment in which the patient lives will profoundly influence the patient's presentation, course of illness, and response (or lack of response) to treatment interventions. It is important, for example, to inquire as to where the patient lives and with whom. Is the patient homeless? Does she have supportive family members at home who can monitor her condition and assist with compliance with mediations and clinic visits? Does she live with people with whom she is in constant conflict and who may serve to destabilize her condition when she leaves the hospital? Is she employed, or will financial strain make it difficult or impossible for her to purchase the particular medication you have just recommended? Without knowledge of this type about a patient's social situation, it would be difficult or impossible to provide the most effective treatment recommendations.

Mistake **#29**

Stumbling through the mental status exam

Assessing the mental status of a patient can be done smoothly and with finesse that is sure to impress your attending. You may complete the mental status exam at the end of your interview, by transitioning with a statement such as, "Now I'd like to ask you some questions to test your thinking and memory." Alternatively, you may weave the mental status exam into your conversation with the patient. For instance, if the patient mentions problems with attention and memory, you may take that opportunity to test these aspects of their mental status. This approach should be used with patients with whom you have built a rapport and can help insure that you don't forget these exams later.

Success Tip #14
Try to incorporate elements of the mental status exam into your conversation with the patient, which will make the interview flow smoothly.

Mistake **#30**

Not recognizing cognitive dysfunction

During the course of any interview, it may become obvious that the patient is not making sense. There are a number of reasons for mental status to be altered, and it is important to inquire about the cognitive functioning of such a patient right away. Once you come to suspect cognitive dysfunction, go ahead and assess the patient's orientation and ability to concentrate and maintain attention. This technique will help you to determine if the patient is delirious or demented. If this is the case, not only will you need to change your interview style, but you will also need to try to determine if the cognitive dysfunction is reversible and begin the appropriate treatment. Missing a diagnosis of delirium may result in the patient's death, so it is important to address this immediately.

Success Tip #15

Delirium must be identified quickly so that investigation and treatment of the underlying illness can be initiated. Delirium is a sign of a dying brain, so a rapid diagnosis is essential.

Mistake #31

Terminating the interview ineffectively

Part of a successful interview is being able to end on time and in a way that is non-injurious to the patient. Especially in team rounds, you will have a certain amount of time to gather all of the necessary information. By following the above guidelines, you will have started with open-ended questions and then narrowed your focus to gather the important information in an empathic way. You should let the patient know that your time is up by thanking them for answering all of your questions and giving them the opportunity to ask you questions. In a team interview, give the rest of the team members an opportunity to ask questions as well. Finally, you should stand up with the patient and escort them to the door.

Success Tip #16
Ending each interview on time will help team rounds run smoothly and show that you are able to maintain control of the interview.

Mistake **#32**

Not knowing how to structure a consult-liaison service interview

The interviewing techniques discussed thus far in this chapter work best for patients on an inpatient psychiatry service. Interviewing patients in an emergency setting or while on a consult-liaison service presents certain difficulties not yet discussed. These patients may be located in a general emergency center or semi-private hospital room, both settings that may make it difficult to conduct a private interview. If possible, take the patient into a private conference room or empty waiting area for the interview. If this is not possible, let the patient know in advance that there may be several team members present. Draw a curtain if possible. If patients hesitate to answer especially sensitive questions, let them know that it is all right. They may prefer to answer them later, if there is more privacy, or to write the answers on a sheet of paper so that their roommates can't hear. Try to be sensitive to helping the patient maintain privacy in this difficult interview setting.

Mistake **#33**

Not using an interpreter when necessary

You are likely to encounter patients whose primary language is not the same as your own. Unlike in other medical specialties where a rudimentary grasp of the language may be sufficient to communicate with patients, the psychiatric interview requires that both parties speak the language fluently. Many of the nuances that are so important in psychiatry will be lost if you are not able to communicate effectively with the patient. Therefore, it is important that you request an interpreter when interviewing patients who speak a language in which you are not fluent.

When interviewing a patient with an interpreter, situate yourself so that you are facing the patient. Direct the question to the patient and observe the patient answering your questions. Be sure to ask the interpreter to tell you exactly what the patient is saying, rather than paraphrasing. Also, ask the interpreter whether the patient is making sense in general. This will help you with your mental status exam. Be sure to note that the interview was conducted with an interpreter when writing up the evaluation.

Chapter 3

Commonly Made Mistakes During

Prerounds

As with many medical fields, during your psychiatry clerkship, you will begin each day by prerounding. You will need to get to the hospital early in the morning before team rounds or attending rounds begin so that you will have time to meet with each of your patients on your own and check on their progress since the day before. You will present this information to your attending and the team during rounds, and it will be used to formulate a plan for the remainder of your patients' course of treatment. In this chapter we will discuss mistakes commonly made during prerounds.

Mistake #34

Setting aside too little time for prerounds

You will need to allocate enough time to see each of your patients and familiarize yourself with what has happened since you last saw them. The amount of time necessary to accomplish these tasks will vary based upon a number of factors. You will probably need more time early in the rotation because you will be less familiar with the rotation and its responsibilities. As you become more comfortable with the rotation, you will probably become more efficient and need less time for prerounding. You will also need to consider the number of patients you are following and the complexity of each patient. Though the actual time needed for each patient may vary considerably, you should allocate at least twenty minutes per patient initially. Of course, you should spend further time talking with your patients later in the day, so focus your prerounding time toward discussing how they did overnight, whether their symptoms have changed, and how they are tolerating their medications. By setting aside enough time to preround, you will be well-prepared to present your patients during rounds.

Mistake #35

Not having a plan for prerounds

Your prerounding plan will depend largely on the type of service on which you are rotating. If you are on a consult-liaison service, you may have patients on different floors of the hospital, or even in different hospitals. In this case, you will need to determine the most efficient route to take. Ideally, you should not retrace your steps, and you should end up where your team meets for rounds. If your patients are all on one unit, you may need to take into consideration their morning schedules. For instance, many inpatient psychiatry units have a certain time for patients to eat their breakfast, shower and complete their grooming and hygiene tasks. You will need to plan accordingly so that you aren't trying to interview your patients while they are trying to get their morning shower.

Success Tip #17
Plan your prerounding route according to where your patients are located, taking into consideration their morning schedules. Try to leave enough time to deal with the unexpected.

Mistake **#36**

Not knowing what to do during prerounds

The goal of prerounds is to familiarize yourself with any events that have occurred since you last saw your patients. You will also need to ascertain whether your patients are improving and whether they are nearing discharge. Review your plan for the day and determine if any of the information you gathered while prerounding would change the plan. Your attending will expect you to know your patients thoroughly, and the information you collect on prerounds will help you shine on rounds.

Mistake **#37**

Failure to review the chart

Your patients' care will continue around the clock, and much may happen while you are away. The chart is a good place to begin in determining what has happened with your patients overnight. The patients' medical conditions may deteriorate or improve. Your resident(s) or attending may work with your patients after you have left. Consultants may leave new recommendations in the chart. Physicians covering during the night may be called to see your patients and change current treatments or implement new treatment interventions. Each of these events should have been documented in the progress notes and/or physician orders sections of the chart, both of which you will need to review each morning.

Mistake #38

Neglecting to speak with hospital staff

One of the most important tasks of your prerounds each day will be to talk with the hospital staff. The nurses who spent the night caring for your patient will have a tremendous amount of helpful information about your patient, information that you will likely miss if you do not ask for it. Inquire with unit staff as to which nurse cared for your patient overnight, or which nurse took report that morning from the nurse who worked the night shift. Ask this nurse how your patient did overnight, and you will gain important information for treating your patient and also impress your team with your initiative and attention to detail. Find out how your patient handled visiting hours and whether there were any behavioral problems that were not documented elsewhere. Additional staff such as technicians, sitters, and clinicians from other disciplines will also be helpful in this manner. Psychiatric patients often present to the doctors one way and to the staff in an entirely different way. By keeping the lines of communication open with the staff, you will gain important information that may help with your diagnosis and treatment plan.

Success Tip #18
Patients may not be able to tell you everything that happened overnight, so review the chart and talk to staff members each morning.

Mistake **#39**

Not keeping up with labs or studies ordered

By checking the physician orders section of the chart, you will know what labs or studies were ordered for your patient. Be sure that you check the chart or computer for results of these studies. Remember that some studies take a few days, so make sure you continue checking for results. If you can't find the results, find out why. Was the study completed? Did the patient refuse? If the study or blood draw was completed, you may be able to call the lab or radiology department, for example, and get the results before they are posted. You may also be able to review radiologic films with the radiologist before rounds, which is sure to impress your attending. It is always a good idea to leave a little extra time in your prerounding schedule to go the "extra mile."

Mistake **#40**

Failure to note whether PRN medications were administered

Patients on psychiatric units or general medical or surgical wards will often have medications ordered to be administered by the nursing staff only as needed, or PRN. Medications for insomnia, agitation, psychosis, anxiety, withdrawal symptoms, pain, or many other conditions may be ordered in this way. You will need to check each morning to see how many doses (if any) of these PRN medications were actually given. This information may be found in various places depending on the routines of your unit. You may find this information in the chart, in nurses' notes, or in the paper or computerized medication administration records. Of course, you may always ask the patient's nurse what medications were recently given, but this type of information is routinely documented as well, and the nurse will also be able to tell you where it is documented. You may wish to look back over several days' worth of medication administration records to track the history of administration of a particular medication and note any trends in use. For instance, if you recognize that your patient becomes agitated and requires PRN medication every afternoon, you may suggest to the team that a medication be ordered to be given routinely.

Mistake #41

Assuming that all ordered medications were taken

For various reasons, psychiatric patients may refuse to take their routinely ordered psychotropic medications. It is crucial that you know if your patient is regularly complying with the treatment you have ordered. The patients may not tell you that they have refused their medications, so you will need to check the chart or medication administration records (as described above) to verify that patients are actually taking their regularly ordered medications.

Success Tip #19
Knowing the status of studies ordered and whether the patient is compliant with medications ordered will send the message that you are the patient's primary clinician. This will undoubtedly impress your attending.

Mistake **#42**

Repeating your initial interview every day

Your daily interview of patients should focus on what is pertinent for that particular patient. The treatment plan devised by the team will include target symptoms, and these should be your focus in your prerounds interview with your patient. You will also want to inquire about how the patient feels he or she is doing—feeling better, the same, or worse? Ask the patient whether he or she is taking his medications, if there are any side effects, and how the medication is helping.

For patients on an inpatient unit, ask about their experience on the unit. Are they participating in groups and tending to their grooming and self-care? Are they eating meals in the common area or spending most of their time in their room? For patients on a consult service, ask about the treatment they are receiving for their medical illness and whether they are participating in treatments such as physical therapy.

Your focused mental status exam should also include the pertinent points for a particular patient. You will not need to ask a depressed patient orientation questions each day, as you would with a delirious patient. As a rule, you should assess safety with every patient every day. Be sure to ask about thoughts of wanting to hurt himself or others and whether he can let staff know if he feels like acting on these thoughts. The information you gather will aid the team in determining the proper precautions that need to be taken with each patient.

Mistake #43

Losing information gathered during prerounds

If you preround successfully using the tips above, you will have gathered a great deal of information about each of your patients. This information will be presented to your team and then written down in the patients' progress notes. Be sure to write down all of the information collected as you preround, as you will likely forget something if you don't. Try to organize the information so that it is readily available to you during your presentation.

Mistake #44

Not giving yourself enough time to gather your thoughts before rounds

Now that you have collected all of the necessary information and jotted it down in an organized fashion, take a few moments to assimilate all of the information and gather your thoughts. You will need to come up with an assessment and plan for each patient, taking into consideration all of the information collected during prerounds. Be sure to leave enough time to formulate your assessment and plan before rounds, and think about recommendations regarding management of your patients.

Mistake **#45**

Not speaking with your resident before rounds

Unlike some of your other core clerkships, in psychiatry work rounds with the resident prior to attending rounds may not be standard operating procedure. If there is a resident on your team, though, you will want to be certain at least to speak briefly with him or her before rounds begin to be sure that you are both up to date and on the same page regarding your patients.

A team that is not synchronized regarding their patients' status during rounds gives an unprofessional appearance and casts doubt upon the quality of management the patients are receiving. A discrepancy of this sort may cast doubt upon your performance as well. Also, reviewing your understanding of the patients' progress and your ideas for further patient management with your resident is a good way to polish your presentation before you present to your attending. The residents may even prepare you for questions they know your attending is likely to put to you during rounds. When the team looks good, you look good, and your grade will reflect this.

Success Tip #20

Write down all of the information you gather during prerounds and use it to formulate your assessment and plan. Speak with your resident before rounds to make sure that you are both on the same page regarding your patients.

Chapter 4

Commonly Made Mistakes

On Call

During your psychiatry clerkship, it is likely that you will spend some time on call. This may be in an emergency department or admissions unit of a psychiatric hospital. Though there will be differences in the call requirements at various institutions, a number of factors remain consistent. Though being on call can be fatiguing, students usually find it enjoyable because they are able to see psychiatric illness presenting in its most acute state. The mistakes commonly made by students on call are reviewed in this chapter.

Mistake **#46**

Being unsure of your call responsibilities

Regardless of whether you have been on call during other clerkships, unfamiliarity with the expectations of psychiatry call is to be expected. It will be very helpful to check with your resident and attending to learn what is expected of you when you are on call. Depending on your institution, you may be on call all night or only for an evening shift. You may be expected to see patients as they arrive for the entire call shift, or you may be required to see only a certain number of patients.

Typically, you will be expected to see new patients and perform a complete psychiatric interview, as reviewed in Chapter 2. You will likely present your findings to your resident or attending and then write an initial evaluation note, detailing your findings and recommendations.

Mistake #47

Not being adequately prepared for your call

There are a number of things that you can do to reduce the stress of your first call on your psychiatry clerkship. Find out beforehand about your on call responsibilities (see Mistake #46). Additionally, come prepared on the day of your call with items you will need for the duration of your call. Most students, interns, and residents who are on call frequently find it helpful to have an on call bag that can be brought to the hospital for each call. You should bring a change of clothes and personal hygiene items if you will be on call overnight. You may also want to bring snacks with you, as you may not have time to get food from the hospital cafeteria before it closes. Finally, bring any books or resources that you will need for interviewing and formulating diagnoses and plans for the patients that you will see or for studying during down time. Frequently, you will be taking over for a student who works on the day shift in the emergency center or admissions department. If possible, arrive a few minutes early to talk with that student, as they will be able to tell you about the routine of the unit.

Success Tip #21
Find out from your resident or attending what will be expected of you while on call and come prepared with any items you will need for your call.

Mistake #48

Essential patient information is not obtained before the patient is seen

Before you see a patient, be sure to have the patient's name, medical record number, and location in the hospital (e.g., psychiatry emergency department, medical/surgical emergency department or psychiatry unit). You can obtain this information from the resident when you are assigned the patient to evaluate and use it to access the patient's medical record and other important information, such as lab studies and imaging test results. Psychiatry emergency departments may keep separate records for patients that are frequently seen that may include the patient's guardianship information, diagnosis, prior admissions, and potential for violence and aggression. Knowing the reason for the patient's evaluation (i.e., auditory hallucinations or suicidality) is also very helpful because you can review your textbooks if necessary before seeing the patient. This will help you know what to ask when obtaining the patient's history.

Mistake #49

Not talking with team members before seeing the patient

After reviewing the patient's available records, you should talk with the nurse who has completed the nursing assessment. You will then have a better idea of the patient's mental status and know whether there is a potential for violence. If you are in a psychiatric emergency department or psychiatric hospital admissions department, there may also be psychiatric technicians who will be able to give you information about their observations of the patient. If you or anyone else is concerned about a patient's potential for violence, ask a staff member to accompany you during the interview.

Success Tip #22

Review available information and talk with staff before seeing the patient in order to get a better idea of what to expect. If there is concern about a patient's potential for violence, ask a staff member to accompany you during the interview.

Mistake #50

Patient is not seen in a timely fashion

Once a patient has been assigned to you and you have obtained information from the medical record and team members, see the patient as soon as possible. The resident or attending will be waiting on you to complete your evaluation so that you can discuss the case and determine the treatment plan.

Mistake #51

Not formulating an assessment and plan before presenting the patient

Most students do a good job of gathering information and presenting the facts of the case to the resident or attending. Superb students also think about the information that they have gathered and try to formulate a differential diagnosis, assessment and plan. This will impress your resident and attending, who will also be evaluating your thought process and problem-solving skills.

Success Tip #23

Attempt to formulate an assessment and plan before presenting the patient to your resident or attending.

Mistake **#52**

Not understanding the primary decision required in emergency setting evaluations

Your on call duty during many of your other clerkships will be to admit those patients that someone else has deemed appropriate for hospitalization. In most institutions, the psychiatrist on call, along with the student on call, will be determining whether the patient meets criteria for inpatient psychiatric hospitalization. The question of disposition is usually the central question that you will be answering on call. You will be determining whether to admit or discharge a patient from the emergency center.

With each patient you evaluate, you will need to decide whether care will be most appropriately managed on an outpatient basis or whether the patient requires psychiatric hospitalization. Typically, this decision will hinge upon whether or not the patient poses an imminent threat to the safety of himself or others.

Success Tip #24

The primary purpose of an emergency center evaluation is to determine whether the patient requires inpatient hospitalization.

Mistake **#53**

Mistaking on call work for outpatient work

When seeing a patient in an emergency setting, management decisions will be made differently than they might in an outpatient office. The clinician evaluating a patient in an on call setting is unlikely to see that patient again. The patient will likely be referred back to their treating psychiatrist or referred to a community mental health clinic. Because of the difficulties in arranging follow-up care from an emergency room, management interventions will differ from those performed in settings where long term follow-up is possible. Initiation of long-term medications, especially those requiring laboratory monitoring, is typically avoided because the practitioner is unable to observe outcomes and monitor response to treatment. Prescribing potential substances of abuse is likewise avoided.

Remember, the primary focus of an emergency setting evaluation is to determine whether the patient requires inpatient hospitalization. Further care needs to be handled in an outpatient setting where continuity of care is possible.

Mistake #54

Failure to appreciate the complexities of suicidality in the emergency setting

You already know that you must ask every patient about suicidality (see Mistake #24). A large number of patients seen on call in an emergency setting will be experiencing suicidal ideation or may have even attempted suicide prior to their presentation. These patients may at times be reluctant to reveal their suicidal thoughts or discuss the extent of their suicidal intention and planning. Alternatively, other patients may present to an emergency setting and feign suicidal intent for a wide variety of reasons. Assessing suicidality in the emergency setting requires an investigation as to the nature of the suicidal thoughts, whether the patient has a plan, and whether there is an intention or a wish to die.

This complex assessment takes many years to master, so you will not be expected to make such a determination on your own. However, because you will be seeing suicidal patients in whatever specialty you choose, you should take this opportunity to observe upper level residents and attending physicians in assessing suicidal patients, and ask them about their thought process in determining the treatment plan.

Success Tip #25
Observe your upper-level resident and attending when they assess suicidal patients and ask them to discuss their rationale for their treatment plan.

Mistake **#55**

Not understanding grounds for involuntary commitment

Patients seen on call in psychiatric practice will disagree at times with the recommendation for inpatient hospitalization for the optimal delivery of their care. In such cases, involuntary hospitalization or commitment may be considered. However, not all patients for whom inpatient care would be the best option may be committed to a psychiatric hospital against their will. Typically, in order to be considered appropriate for involuntary commitment, a patient must pose a direct threat to the safety of self or others or generally be unable to care for himself. These impairments must also be considered to be the result of psychiatric illness. Additionally, patients suffering from psychiatric illness may develop impairment of judgment resulting from their illness which may render them incapable of making reasoned decisions regarding their treatment. Because these patients cannot give informed consent for inpatient hospitalization, they too should be committed.

Mistake **#56**

Forgetting to investigate thoroughly for substance abuse

Along with an assessment of suicidality, every patient must be asked directly about substance abuse. A large percentage of psychiatric emergency presentations are influenced by substance abuse, and this issue will certainly influence treatment decisions and may factor significantly in the decision to discharge or admit a patient for psychiatric hospitalization. Patients dealing with substance abuse or dependence may, for various reasons, be reluctant to reveal this information. Thus, each patient in need of emergent psychiatric evaluation must be screened thoroughly for substance abuse, ideally both in the psychiatric interview as well as by urine toxicology screening.

Mistake #57

Missing the big picture

When you are learning to deal with emergency center visits, you can easily fall into the routine of simply gathering information along a strict H&P route and focusing largely on psychiatric symptoms. While this type of information is essential, one must not lose sight of the forest for the trees. There are some specific big picture issues to keep in mind when evaluating patients on call in an emergency setting. Why did the patient choose this particular time to report to the emergency center? How did the patient get to the EC? Did he walk, or take the bus, or drive himself? Did a friend or family member persuade the patient to report to the EC and take him there? Were police or emergency services involved, and if so, who called them? What exactly does the patient hope to gain from the visit? Where and with whom does he live? Who provides support for the patient? What does he plan to do if discharged from the emergency center? Each of these questions is part of the big picture and can be quite useful when assessing patients on call, even aiding in determining whether a patient should be discharged or admitted to a psychiatric hospital.

Success Tip #26
Remember to look at the big picture while assessing each patient in an emergency setting.

Mistake **#58**

Not obtaining collateral information

Frequently patients will be unable to provide a reliable history. It will be important that you attempt to contact family members who may be able to provide the information that you need. If the patient lives in a care home, call the facility and speak with the patient's caregivers. You may also be able to get medical record information from other facilities in which the patient has been recently. Your residents will greatly appreciate your efforts in gathering this collateral information. It will leave them with more time to teach and prepare you for attending rounds.

Mistake **#59**

Discussing with the patient or family issues about which you are unsure

Medical students often spend more time with patients and their families than any other member of the team. Naturally, they may ask students specific questions about the treatment plan or prognosis of the patient. You should generally defer these questions to your resident or attending. It is never appropriate for you to give information about which you are unsure. Rather, let them know that you will discuss their questions with the team. Be sure that you then go with the resident or attending when they discuss these questions with the patient, as this will be a good learning experience. Also, remember that confidentiality is important, even in an emergency center (see Mistake #15).

Mistake **#60**

Leaving all of the paperwork and orders for the resident to write

Once the team has decided to admit a patient, there will be a significant amount of paperwork to do. You should be as involved as possible in filling out admission paperwork, admission orders, and commitment papers. Once again, your resident will be appreciative for your help, and you will better understand the treatment plan for the patient. The resident will need to review the orders and papers with you and co-sign them.

The following table contains the standard elements of the psychiatric admission orders.

Psychiatric admission orders

Element	What to write
Admit to	Psychiatry unit, team, attending
Status	Voluntary or involuntary
Diagnosis	Axis I, II, and III diagnoses
Condition	Good/fair/satisfactory
Vital Signs	q day is usually sufficient for most patients on psychiatry units, unless the patient has medical problems or withdrawal symptoms that require more frequent monitoring
Allergies	List drug allergies here; if there are no drug allergies, write NKDA which stands for no known drug allergy
Activity	Unit restriction, precautions and checks for suicidality, agitation, elopement, etc. Also indicate if the patient is allowed to smoke per unit protocol
Nursing	Instructions for nursing care may include fingerstick glucose measurements, wound care/dressing changes, etc
Diet	Regular, renal diet, ADA diet for DM, low-sodium, low-protein, lactose-restricted
Consults	Social Work and Occupational Therapy for evaluation and therapy
Medications	Specify the medication as well as the dosage, frequency, and route of administration; include PRN medications for agitation if indicated
Labs	Specify when and what type of laboratory tests should be ordered
Special	Include anything else here that you haven't listed above

Chapter 5

Commonly Made Mistakes On

Write-Ups

The write-up or written case presentation is a detailed account of the patient's clinical presentation. Your write-ups will be placed in the medical record, along with those of the resident and attending. Additionally, you may be required to turn one or more write-ups in to your attending as part of your grade. Besides testing your knowledge of psychiatry, the write-up also helps you develop written communication skills. Being able to communicate patient information in an organized and succinct way, either orally or written, will be important throughout your medical career. This chapter focuses on mistakes students commonly make on write-ups.

Mistake #61

Not understanding the importance of the write-up

The write-ups that you turn in will be reviewed by your attending and perhaps your clerkship director, and they may play a large role in the determination of your overall grade for the clerkship. The write-ups that go in the chart become a part of the patient's medical record. The student write-up is often the most detailed document in the chart, so physicians and staff will likely reference it for years to come. For this reason, it is important that you are careful to be accurate.

Success Tip #27

Write-ups play a large role in the determination of
your overall grade and become a part of the
patient's "permanent (medical) record," so be
sure that your write-up is an accurate and high-
quality document.

Mistake **#62**

The write-up is not turned in on time

If you are turning in your write-up to your attending, be
sure it is on time. Turning in your write-up late will likely
result in a lower grade. Turning your write-up in on time
will also allow the attending to give you feedback that will
help you prepare for the next write-up. If the write-up is
going in the chart, place it there as soon as possible so
that the information is available to other clinicians.

Mistake **#63**

Not knowing what to include in the write-up

You will want to talk with your attending or clerkship
director to find out what they want included in your write-
up. However, there are some basic elements that you will
likely need to include in your write-up. This is also the
preferred order in which your write-up should be
organized. Write-ups that do not adhere to the expected
order are considered disorganized and difficult to follow.
Your write-up should include the following:

49

- Chief complaint
- Reason for consultation and referral source (for consults only)
- History of present illness (HPI)
- Review of psychiatric symptoms
- Past psychiatric history
- Past medical and surgical history (PMH/PSH)
- Medications
- Medication allergies
- Family history (especially family psychiatric history)
- Social and developmental history
- Mental status exam (include MMSE, clock drawing if indicated)
- Review of systems and physical exam (if indicated)
- Laboratory data
- Other studies (e.g., head CT, MRI, EEG)
- Biopsychosocial formulation
- Differential diagnosis
- DSM-IV multiaxial diagnoses
- Biopsychosocial treatment plan

Success Tip #28
Make sure you include all of the elements expected in your write-up and that it is organized in the correct format.

Mistake #64

The date and time of the assessment is not included in the write-up

The date and time must be on every document in the medical record. Likewise, put the date and time on the write-up turned in to your attending. You need to get into this habit early.

Mistake #65

The source of the history is not included

Often history will be gathered from sources other than the patient. This may include family, friends, caretakers and the medical record. In addition to indicating who provided the history, note the reliability of the source. Including the informant's phone number can also be very helpful.

Success Tip #29
Indicate the source of the information in the evaluation, and comment on the reliability of that source.

Mistake #66

Not using the history to present a case for your assessment

The write-up should not be a mere list of symptoms, nor should it be a word-for-word account of the patient's story. An inventory of the patient's complaints in his own words and a review of symptomatology from the main diagnostic categories of psychiatric disease are essential components of the evaluation. However, this information must be presented in the write-up in a clearly organized fashion so that the reader is able to discern the main themes of the case presentation leading up to the assessment and plan. You can think of the assessment as the argument you are making for a specific diagnostic picture, and the body of the write-up should contain the supporting information for the argument you are presenting. Thus, the chief complaint, history of present illness, past psychiatric and medical history, family history, social and developmental histories, and the mental status exam and diagnostic studies function as parts of a whole and complement one another in their support of the diagnostic "argument" you are making about the case.

Mistake #67

The history of present illness does not flow well

The HPI is a description of why the patient is here now. It is considered to be one of the most important elements of the patient write-up, as it sets the stage for your assessment and plan. The HPI should flow like a story, giving the reader a clear idea of the events that transpired before the patient sought treatment. In order to avoid a disjointed and confusing HPI, present the information in a chronological fashion beginning with when the patient was last at his or her baseline.

Example:

> Mr. Brown is a 35-year-old male with no prior psychiatric history who presents with a 2 month

history of depressed mood, decreased interests, insomnia with early morning awakening, decreased appetite with 10 lb weight loss, low energy, poor concentration, tearfulness, and thoughts that life is not worth living. He identifies no precipitant for these symptoms.

Success tip #30
The HPI should tell the story of how the patient came to be evaluated by you and set the stage for your assessment and diagnosis.

HPI checklist

Use the following checklist to make sure your HPI has been well constructed:

☐ HPI identifies the time of symptom onset

☐ HPI includes duration of symptoms

☐ HPI traces development of symptoms from onset to the current time (chronological)

☐ HPI addresses why the patient has sought medical/psychiatric attention now

☐ Precipitants of the patient's symptom(s) are included (e.g., death or illness in family, marital problem, relationship problem [family, significant other, friend], medical illness, work difficulties, stressful events at school, financial difficulties, legal problem, anniversary of negative event, medication noncompliance, substance abuse, other stresses/changes)

☐ HPI includes factors that alleviate the patient's symptoms

☐ Pertinent features of the past psychiatric history are included in the HPI

☐ Pertinent features of the past medical or surgical history are included in the HPI (i.e., current illness or previous surgery that is contributing or accounting for the patient's symptoms)

☐   Pertinent features of the family history are included in the HPI

☐   Pertinent features of the sexual history are included in the HPI

☐   Review of systems that is pertinent to the chief complaint is included in the HPI

☐   HPI includes patient's concerns, fears, and thoughts about what may be accounting for his or her symptoms

☐   The degree to which the psychiatric illness is affecting the patient's functioning is included (baseline and current functioning with regards to relationships with family/significant other/friends, occupation, school, and leisure activities)

Mistake #68

Too many abbreviations are used

Many physicians use copious abbreviations and acronyms in their write-ups, which make them difficult to read and interpret. While there may be some abbreviations and acronyms that are ubiquitous (e.g., HTN for hypertension or SI for suicidal ideations), many are specific to the physician and institution. When a physician in another community reads the medical record, he or she may not be sure what the abbreviations mean. This may result in treatment errors. In fact, some abbreviations and shorthand used in writing prescriptions have been outlawed by the hospital accreditation agency in order to avoid medication errors. As a rule of thumb, avoid using abbreviations and acronyms as much as possible.

With regard to your HPI, be sure to write in complete sentences, rather than using abbreviations or short phrases. Remember that you are telling a story in the HPI, so it should read like one.

Mistake **#69**

Drawing conclusions in the HPI

The HPI should be what the patient reports, in the patient's own words as much as possible. Do not draw conclusions or make diagnoses in the HPI. For example, you should write, "The patient reported depressed mood, decreased interests, insomnia, decreased appetite and low energy" rather than "The patient reported symptoms of depression."

Mistake **#70**

Review of major psychiatric symptoms is not included

As a separate section, or at the end of your HPI, document pertinent positive and negative symptoms for major psychiatric disorders, including depression, mania, psychosis, anxiety, and eating disorders. If the patient uses alcohol or drugs, be sure to note that in the HPI, including whether there is a history of withdrawal symptoms, blackouts, seizures, delirium tremens, etc. If the patient does not use alcohol or drugs, this should be noted in this section or in the social history section. Sample questions that can be used to screen for the major psychiatric disorders are included in the interview template in Appendix F.

Example:

> Mr. Brown often worries about things that are out of his control but denies other anxiety disorder symptoms. He denies current or previous symptoms of racing thoughts, decreased need for sleep, grandiosity, hallucinations, or

delusions. He has never smoked or used drugs.
He drinks three or four beers a day. He has had
some mild tremors when he cuts back on his
drinking. He has never had withdrawal seizures
or DTs.

Success Tip #31

The review of major psychiatric symptoms allows
the clinician to narrow the differential diagnosis by
ruling out other conditions.

Checklist for review of psychiatric symptoms

Your review of psychiatric symptoms is complete if you
have included (or excluded) the following:

- ☐ Symptoms of Mood Disorders
- ☐ Symptoms of Psychotic Disorders
- ☐ Symptoms of Anxiety Disorders
- ☐ Symptoms of Substance Use Disorders
- ☐ Symptoms of Cognitive Disorders

Mistake #71

The past psychiatric history is not complete

The past psychiatric history should contain information
about current clinicians (psychiatrist, therapist, case
manager) and when they were last seen, hospitalization
history, suicide attempt history, self-mutilation history,
and psychiatric medication history. Not all patients will be
able to provide all of this information, so look for collateral
sources of information such as the medical record,

summaries from previous and current clinicians, and family or friends. The absence of any of these aspects of the history should also be noted.

Success Tip #32

The past psychiatric history should include information about current clinicians, prior hospitalizations, prior suicide attempts, self-mutilation, and medication trials.

Checklist for past psychiatric history

Your psychiatrist history is complete if you have included the following:

☐ Names and contact information of current clinicians (psychiatrist, therapist, psychopharmacologist, social worker, group therapist, primary care physician)

☐ Dates of last and next appointments with current clinicians

☐ Prior hospitalizations (psychiatric/chemical dependency), including age at first hospitalization, total number, reasons for hospitalization, location, voluntary/involuntary status, and date of last hospitalization

☐ Suicide attempt history, including number of attempts, methods, and lethality

☐ Self-mutilation history, including why the patient mutilates and the effect

☐ Psychiatric medications taken by patient in the past, including indications for each medication, response, any adverse reactions, maximum dosages reached, and duration of treatment

Mistake #72

The past medical and surgical history is not complete

Be sure to list all of the patient's medical problems, including current treatments and status of the problem. For illnesses that contribute to psychiatric illness or inform treatment, such as head trauma, seizure disorders, diabetes mellitus, liver disease, etc., note negative history as well. You should also include past obstetric/gynecologic and surgical history, as well as significant childhood illnesses here.

Checklist for PMSH

Your past medical and surgical history is complete if you have included the following:

☐　All current and past medical problems, including current treatments and status of illness (active, well-controlled, remission)

☐　Presence or absence of head trauma (include loss of consciousness, need for hospitalization, resultant deficits), seizure disorders, liver disease, thyroid disease, diabetes mellitus

☐　Surgical history and obstetric/gynecologic history

☐　Significant childhood illnesses

Mistake #73

Medication list is not complete

List all the prescription medications that the patient is taking, as well as over-the-counter medications and herbal supplements. Be sure to note the patient's

compliance with prescribed medications. Many over-
the-counter medications and supplements contain
psychoactive ingredients that may be playing a role in
the current symptoms, so don't overlook this important
part of the history. Patients may forget to tell you about
them, so be sure to ask specifically. Many herbal
preparations contain more than one supplement, so ask
the patient to bring in the bottle in order to get a
complete list of ingredients. If the patient is not taking
any over-the-counter or herbal medications, note this in
your write-up as well.

Success Tip #33

Be sure to document all prescribed and over-
the-counter medications and any supplements
that the patient is taking. Indicate whether the
patient is compliant with prescribed
medications.

Medication checklist

Your medication list is complete if you have included
the following:

☐ Names of all prescribed medications the patient is
   taking, along with dosage and route of
   administration

☐ Names of all over-the-counter medications the
   patient is taking, along with dosage and route of
   administration

☐ Names of all herbal supplements the patient is
   taking, along with dosage and route of
   administration

☐ Recently discontinued medications followed by
   the notation "recently discontinued" in
   parentheses

Mistake #74

Medication allergies are not described

List all the patient's medication allergies and specify what the allergic reaction is. Often, what a patient considers an allergic reaction is actually a side effect of the medication. For instance, patients often say they are allergic to Haldol because it makes them stiff. This is not an allergy, but the common side effect of EPS (extra-pyramidal symptoms). If a patient does not have any medication allergies, write "NKDA."

Mistake #75

The family history is not complete

Some attendings may ask that you draw a family pedigree, incorporating any illness that the family members may have. Others simply want a list of close family members and their illnesses. On your psychiatry rotation, you should focus especially on the family psychiatric history. The heritability of many psychiatric illnesses has been well established, and a family history of specific psychiatric disorders or intergenerational suicides may aid in establishing a diagnosis. Include family members' diagnoses, treatment, hospitalizations, and suicide attempts and completions. While you should try to include the full medical family history as well, focus especially on illnesses with psychiatric manifestations (i.e., thyroid disease, multiple sclerosis, seizure disorder, etc.) and illnesses that might dictate treatment choices (i.e., sudden cardiac death, arrhythmias, hepatic disease, etc.).

Success Tip #34
The family history section should include all psychiatric diagnoses, medications, and suicide attempts or completions in the family.

Family history checklist
The following are necessary for your family history to be complete:

☐ Any history of psychiatric illness in biological relatives, including diagnoses, treatment (and whether it was effective), hospitalizations, suicide attempts and completions (include suicide attempts in non-biological relatives as well)

☐ Medical history in biological relatives, focusing on illnesses with psychiatric manifestations (thyroid disease, neurological disease, etc.) and those that might dictate treatment (cardiac disease, hepatic disease, renal disease, diabetes mellitus, etc.)

Mistake **#76**

The social history is not complete

In psychiatry, the social history is one of the major parts of the write-up because a patient's environment can play a significant role in the development and treatment of psychiatric illness. Include a description of current and prior relationships (parents, siblings, spouse/partner, children, and friends), living situation, education, occupation, disability status, legal history, abuse history and sexual history. Remember to include any information relevant to the presenting problem in the HPI.

Example:

> Mr. Brown lives in a home with his wife of ten years and two children, ages 8 and 4. He describes his wife as supportive and feels that they have a good marriage. He enjoys his children whom he describes as good kids. He completed a bachelor's degree at the state university and works as a high school math teacher, which he enjoys but finds very stressful. He denies any legal history. He grew up in a small rural community and has one younger sister, with whom he gets along well. His father, a banker, was "distant" and uninvolved with the children growing up. He drank heavily and died of cirrhosis of the liver several years ago. His mother was a teacher, and he felt very close to her growing up. He denies any history of physical, emotional, or sexual abuse. He is heterosexual, began dating at age 17 and was first sexually active at age 19. He has never been arrested or incarcerated.

Success Tip #35

The social history is very important in psychiatry and should include a description of significant relationships, living situation, education, occupation, disability status, legal history, abuse history, and sexual history.

Checklist for social history

Your social history is complete if you have included the following:

☐   Where the patient was born and raised

☐   Performance in school and extent of education

☐   Occupation and employment status (if not currently employed, has patient ever been employed?)

☐   Disability status

☐   Legal history (including incarcerations, arrests, probation/parole status)

☐   History of physical, emotional, sexual abuse

☐   Sexual history

☐   Relationships with parents, siblings, spouse/ partner, children, friends

☐   Any current stressors (may also be included in HPI)

Mistake **#77**

The mental status exam is not complete

In the HPI, use the patient's words to describe his subjective experience. In the mental status exam (MSE), use medical terms to describe your observations. The MSE should be thorough but concise. For instance, you should write "paranoid ideations" instead of "the patient thinks someone is after him." By using the proper terminology, you can demonstrate your mastery of the language of psychiatry. Your MSE can be written either in

paragraph form or as a list. Ask your attending what he or
she prefers.

Example:

> Appearance: overweight, well-groomed,
> appeared stated age
> Eye Contact: limited, patient looked at floor often
> Behavior: appropriate, cooperative
> Activity: decreased motor activity
> Speech: paucity of speech, slowed rate, low
> volume, monotone
> Mood: depressed
> Affect: constricted, congruent with mood
> Thought Processes: logical and goal-directed,
> though slowed at times
> Thought Content: thoughts that life's not worth
> living but no suicide plan or intent; no
> homicidality; no delusions or obsessions
> Perceptions: no hallucinations or illusions
> Sensorium: alert, oriented to person, place, and
> time
> Memory: good recent and remote memory
> Concentration: good
> Abstract Thinking: intact, answer to spilled milk
> proverb was, "It is no use to worry about things
> that are out of your control"
> Insight: fairly good, realizes he needs help
> Judgment: good
> Intellect: above average

Mistake #78

Cognitive screening is not noted when indicated

Some attendings may require that you include the mini-
mental status exam (MMSE) for every patient. Be sure to

ask what your attending prefers. If you are not required to do an MMSE for every patient, be sure that you perform this exam on patients with any evidence of cognitive dysfunction, including elderly patients, some depressed patients that report memory problems, and anyone with any history of brain injury, just to name a few. You can also perform a clock drawing test, which tests parts of the brain not tested by the MMSE. The clock drawing test can be especially useful in patients with any type of head injury or evidence of executive dysfunction such as poor planning and execution of tasks, problems with working memory, socially inappropriate behavior, changes in personality, etc. These examinations are detailed in Appendix H.

Success Tip #36
A mental status exam should be noted for every patient, and cognitive screening should be included if there is any evidence of cognitive dysfunction.

MSE checklist

A complete mental status exam should include the following:

☐ Appearance (grooming, hygiene, age, weight, oddities)

☐ Eye contact

☐ Behavior (cooperation, attitude)

☐ Psychomotor activity (decreased, increased, agitated)

☐ Speech (rate, volume, tone, paucity)

☐ Mood (in the patient's words)

☐ Affect (your observation; note congruence with mood and thought content)

☐ Thought processes (logical, goal-directed, circumstantial, tangential, flight of ideas, loose associations, disorganized)

☐ Thought content (delusions, obsessions, suicidal/ homicidal ideations)

☐ Perception (illusions, hallucinations)

☐ Sensorium (level of alertness, orientation, attention/ concentration, memory)

☐ Abstraction

☐ Insight

☐ Judgment

☐ Mini Mental Status Exam and Clock Drawing (if indicated)

Mistake #79

Vital signs are not listed

Every patient presenting to an emergency or admissions department should have vital signs taken. Vital signs may be taken by the nurse or yourself. The vital signs may be the first indication that a patient is intoxicated or withdrawing from a substance or that they have an unstable general medical condition. If you suspect one of these conditions, you should recheck the patient's vital signs to determine if there has been a change in the patient's condition.

Mistake #80

Physical exam is omitted

Patients admitted to an inpatient psychiatry unit should have documentation of a physical examination. Additionally, any patient with psychiatric symptoms that you suspect are secondary to a general medical condition should have a complete physical exam. Since there is significant overlap between psychiatric and neurological illnesses, your neurological examination must be thoroughly documented. Stating that the neurological exam is "non-focal" is inadequate.

Success Tip #37

Vital signs should be taken on every patient and are often the first indicator of a general medical condition. A physical exam, with an especially thorough neurological examination, should be done on all admissions.

Mistake **#81**

Laboratory data is not included

Unless the patient has documentation of recent laboratory data, all patients admitted to the unit and many who present to the emergency center should have basic labs ordered. In addition to aiding in your assessment for general medical conditions, labs are necessary to monitor adverse effects and medication compliance. Be sure that any medication that has an available assay for serum level is ordered and documented. All patients should also have a urine drug screen, and anyone with a history of alcohol use should have an alcohol level. Female patients of child-bearing age should have a urine pregnancy test as well.

Mistake #82

Results of other studies are not reported

The results of any other diagnostic tests should be included in the write-up, such as a head CT, MRI, or EEG. If the patient had an EKG or other radiographs, you may include this information as well. If the official report is not available at the time the write-up is due, you may offer your own interpretation and indicate that the final report is pending.

Success Tip #38
Laboratory data and results of studies should be recorded in the write-up. If they have been ordered but not completed or interpreted, note that they are pending. You may also provide your own interpretation.

Checklist for other data

The following data should also be noted in the write-up:

☐ Physical examination, with thorough neurological examination

☐ Laboratory data (toxicology screen, alcohol level, pregnancy test, serum drug levels, metabolic panel, complete blood count)

☐ Results of diagnostic tests (CT scan, MRI, EEG, EKG, other radiographs)

Mistake #83

Biopsychosocial formulation is not included

The biopsychosocial formulation serves to summarize the salient features of your write-up. It takes into consideration the biological, psychological, and social factors that may be contributing to your patient's current presentation. Many clinicians include spiritual factors as a fourth contributing category. This formulation is a way to tie together the life history and current symptomatology of the patient into a story. In the biological factors section, include such things as personal and family history of psychiatric illness, medical illnesses that may contribute to psychiatric symptoms, and use of any psychoactive medications, drugs or alcohol. The psychological section should include any events, relationships, experiences, etc. that may have shaped the way the patient perceives and copes with stressors. You can include defense mechanisms here. The social factors influencing current symptoms may include any stressors in the patient's environment.

The biopsychosocial formulation is an advanced way of conceptualizing patients and takes a lot of practice to master. However, if you make an effort to include this formulation in your write-up, it will only boost your evaluation. Learning this way of conceptualizing patients will also be useful in your future practice of medicine. It will help you take into consideration the *whole person* of the patient, resulting in improved care.

Example:

> *In summary, Mr. Brown is a 35-year-old gentleman with depressive symptoms and alcohol dependence. Biological factors*

contributing to his alcohol dependence include a genetic predisposition as a result of his father's alcoholism. His own alcohol use may be contributing to his depressive symptoms, along with a family history of depression in his sister. Medical conditions, such as thyroid disease, should be considered as they may also cause depressive symptoms. Psychological factors include the long-term effects of his growing up with an emotionally distant father by whom he never felt valued. He may have turned to alcohol as a way to self-medicate. Further, since he was not able to resolve his feelings toward his father before he died, he is grieving not only the loss of his father, but also the loss of the opportunity for his ideal father-son relationship. The resulting grief may be related to his drinking and depressive symptoms. Though Mr. Brown enjoys his children and describes himself as a good father, he likely fears that he may become his own father, resulting in a distant relationship between him and his children. Mr. Brown's job is stressful and may also be contributing to his current symptoms and need to "unwind" using alcohol.

Success Tip #39

The biopsychosocial formulation is an advanced way of conceptualizing patients that takes into account the whole person and experience of the patient. Practice thinking about all of your patients in this way.

Biopsychosocial formulation checklist

Your biopsychosocial formulation should include the following:

☐   Biological factors contributing to illness (personal and family history of psychiatric illness, medical illness with psychiatric symptoms, psychoactive medications, drugs, alcohol)

☐   Psychological factors contributing to illness (coping strategies, defense mechanisms, relationships, abuse, etc.)

☐   Social factors contributing to illness (occupational/ financial problems, relationships, support system)

☐   Spiritual factors contributing to illness

Mistake #84

Multiaxial DSM diagnoses not listed

When presenting a psychiatric diagnosis, particularly in written form, be sure to standardize your assessment according to the diagnostic gold standard of psychiatry, the Diagnostic and Statistical Manual of Mental Disorders, or DSM. Published and updated periodically by the American Psychiatric Association, the DSM offers a standardized and universally accepted list of psychiatric diagnoses and the criteria by which they are diagnosed. It also presents the Multiaxial Assessment, the system by which practitioners may organize their diagnostic assessment according to five specific domains, or axes, thus facilitating the complex process of evaluating patients and formulating psychiatric treatment plans. The five axes included in the DSM multiaxial system are:

Axis I: Clinical Psychiatric Disorders
Axis II: Personality Disorders
             Mental Retardation
             Developmental Disorders
Axis III: General Medical Conditions
Axis IV: Psychosocial and Environmental
             Stressors
Axis V: Global Assessment of Functioning

You will need to use this method of assessment in your write-ups. Diagnostic criteria for some of the major clinical syndromes are contained in Appendix C, but you will probably also need a DSM for use during your clerkship, which has a complete listing of all diagnostic criteria.

Success Tip #40
Every patient that you see will require a multiaxial assessment, so learn which conditions go on each axis sooner rather than later.

Mistake **#85**

Differential diagnosis is not complete

When considering the differential diagnosis for the patient, it is helpful to think along the lines of the major clinical disorders and provide evidence for or against each diagnostic category. For Axis I disorders, the five major categories are mood disorders, anxiety disorders, psychotic disorders, substance use disorders, and cognitive dysfunction disorders. Remember that many psychiatric symptoms can be secondary to general medical conditions and substance intoxication or withdrawal, so be sure to include these in your differential. Another diagnostic category, especially important in children, is disruptive behavior disorders. For Axis II, think about the personality traits evident in the patient and whether they constitute a personality disorder.

Success Tip #41

Use the information gathered in your review of major psychiatric symptoms as evidence for or against each of the major categories of psychiatric disorders in your differential diagnosis. The information gathered in the social history pertaining to relationships, job performance, and childhood will help you with the differential for personality disorders.

Checklist for diagnosis

Your diagnosis section is complete if you have included the following:

☐   Differential diagnosis (discuss major categories of Axis I disorders and personality disorders on Axis II)
☐   Multiaxial DSM Diagnoses
      Axis I: Clinical Psychiatric Disorders
      Axis II: Personality Disorders
              Mental Retardation
              Developmental Disorders
      Axis III: General Medical Conditions
      Axis IV: Psychosocial and Environmental Stressors
      Axis V: Global Assessment of Functioning

Mistake #86

Neglecting the plan

Medical students often work very thoroughly and logically toward making a case for a diagnosis only to then fall short when it comes to presenting a plan for treating the disorder they have just diagnosed. It can be easy for a student to think that the limited experience of a novice is insufficient to formulate an adequate plan for treatment. Do not fall into this trap. It is very important to make an attempt at formulating a treatment plan for the disorder diagnosed in your write-up. Without this plan, your write-up is incomplete.

Mistake #87

Failing to present a biopsychosocial treatment plan

Your treatment plan must be thorough, addressing all realms of the patient's functioning in a global manner. This is best and most reliably accomplished by developing a treatment plan using the biopsychosocial (spiritual) approach that you used in your formulation. For any patient's disorder, you should think along biological lines, such as prescribing medications that may be indicated, discontinuing medications that may be contributing, treating underlying medical conditions, etc. If the patient requires inpatient hospitalization, be sure to specify this in your treatment plan.

You must also consider a psychological perspective, perhaps selecting a specific type of psychotherapy that is likely to also provide benefit for the patient. Then you will need to analyze the patient's social situation to determine which types of interventions are indicated to provide additional support. Finally, after carefully considering the patient's particular religious and spiritual orientation, you may also choose to implement a spiritual component to the assessment and treatment plan. By thinking along these lines, treatment is ensured to be fully comprehensive.

Success Tip #42

You will need to formulate a treatment plan for each patient you evaluate. You can use the biopsychosocial model to formulate a comprehensive treatment plan that addresses each component of the patient's illness.

Checklist for treatment plan

Your treatment plan should include:

☐   Biological treatments (hospital admission, medications, diagnostic tests, treating underlying medical conditions, discontinuing medications or illicit drugs that may be contributing to illness)

☐   Psychological treatments (psychotherapy)

☐   Social interventions (social services consult to help with any outstanding social needs, referral to support groups)

☐   Spiritual interventions (pastoral consult or counseling)

Chapter 6

Commonly Made Mistakes When

Presenting New Patients

Whether you are rotating in an inpatient unit, a consultation-liaison service, the emergency room, or an outpatient clinic, you will most likely be expected to present new patient evaluations to your attending or team. The purpose of the oral case presentation is to inform the attending physician or team members about the patient. Generally, depending upon the service on which you are rotating, the oral presentation should be a formal one. However, it should also be succinct, without any unnecessary details. This is the main difference between the oral case presentation and the write-up, which includes much more information.

As mentioned in Chapter 5, good communication skills are essential for today's physicians. You must be able to present information clearly and concisely in both written and oral mediums. This chapter focuses on helping students develop their oral presentation skills by discussing mistakes commonly made during oral presentations of new patients.

Mistake **#88**

Underestimating the importance of the oral case presentation

The oral case presentation is one of the most important aspects of your psychiatry rotation. The goal of the oral presentation is to communicate the facts of the patient's presentation to the attending physician or team and to convey your assessment of the patient's clinical status and an outline for treatment. The oral case presentation will thus serve as an example of your ability to evaluate and treat psychiatric patients. Therefore, the quality of your oral case presentations will significantly influence the grade you will receive on your psychiatry rotation.

Success Tip #43
Your attending will determine your ability to evaluate and treat patients based largely upon your oral case presentations.

Mistake **#89**

Not knowing how much time you have to present the case

You will need to verify with your attending how much time you have to present the case, but generally you should take no more than ten to fifteen minutes. This may sound like a lot of time, but it isn't. Many students make the mistake of taking twenty to thirty minutes or more to present a new patient, a sure-fire way to annoy the rest of your team members, who likely have a long "To Do" list. Practice presenting new patients in a timely manner. Your team will thank you for it.

Mistake #90

Not understanding the appropriate order and content of the presentation

The order and content of the oral case presentation will be generally consistent with that of the write-up. Convention dictates that you present the following sections in the following order:

- Chief complaint
- History of present illness
- Past psychiatric history
- Past medical history
- Medications
- Medication allergies
- Family psychiatric history
- Social history
- Developmental history
- Mental status exam
- Vital signs and physical exam
- Laboratory data
- Other diagnostic studies
- Biopsychosocial assessment
- DSM-IV multiaxial assessment
- Biopsychosocial treatment plan

Success Tip #44

Familiarity with the expected order and content of the case presentation will aid you in giving a succinct presentation.

Mistake **#91**

Not appreciating the difference between the write-up and the oral case presentation

While, as mentioned above, much of the content of the case presentation will reproduce the content of the write-up, there are important differences between the two. Most importantly, an oral case presentation should typically be more succinct than a write-up, focusing on the more pertinent details of the case. The goal is to present all material relevant to formulating the diagnosis and establishing appropriate treatment while maintaining the attention of the attending physician and team members. Students commonly make the mistake of being over-inclusive in detail when presenting cases orally, making the presentation too long. Such over-inclusiveness will likely interfere with the attending physician's ability to follow the key points of the case and result in a less impressive presentation.

Mistake **#92**

Reading the oral case presentation

While it may be reassuring to perform an oral case presentation by reading the written history and physical aloud, doing so is certainly a mistake. The oral case presentation is meant to be more succinct than the write-up, conveying very efficiently the key details of the case. By reading your write-up aloud for the oral presentation, you will likely present information that is overly inclusive in detail. Additionally, reading a written case aloud is a sure way to lose the attention of your audience. When presenting, you should keep your audience in mind, making sure that they are tuned in to you.

Though a presentation is by nature rather one sided, your oral case presentation should have a subjective tone that is interactive and dynamic, thereby keeping the audience in tune with you and engaged as you present. You should maintain eye contact with your audience reasonably well during the presentation, conveying a sense of ease with the material and confidence in your performance. It will be difficult if not impossible to accomplish these tasks if you are reading your presentation from a written page.

Success Tip #45

Don't simply read your write-up. Your case presentation should focus on the pertinent details and be delivered in a way that keeps your audience engaged.

Mistake **#93**

Not practicing your oral case presentation with your resident

If you are to present a polished presentation to your attending without reading it, then you must of course first practice. You should take advantage of the opportunity to present your cases first to your resident and receive feedback before presenting to the attending physician. If your residents do not ask you to present the case to them alone beforehand, ask if you may do this for your learning. Residents have a great deal of experience in this arena and will be able to help you improve your presentations significantly, allowing you to shine when you then present to your attending physician.

Mistake #94

Not observing resident presentations closely

As mentioned above, your residents will be well seasoned in the oral presentation of cases. You should observe and learn from their techniques. You will also likely be able to detect preferences the particular attending may have for the oral presentation. Thus, the style of the residents' oral presentations should influence your presentations. Be careful, though, not to copy the resident's style exactly, as there will likely be different expectations for student presentations.

Mistake #95

Not appreciating the expectations for a student presenter

As discussed above, you can learn a lot from listening to residents present cases. However, there are differences in the expectations for a resident presenter and for a student. As is often the case in medicine in general, it is expected that students be more thorough and formal as they are at an early point in the medical education process and benefit greatly from practicing very thorough techniques as they are developing their skills. Thus, the student will likely be expected to be more inclusive in their presentation than the resident.

Success Tip #46
You may get some helpful tips on presentation style by observing residents, but remember that, as a student, you will be expected to give more thorough and formal presentations.

Mistake **#96**

Presenting in an unprofessional manner

The oral case presentation is one of the more formal educational activities students are expected to perform. Nothing will mar a presentation more quickly than an overly informal or unprofessional presentational style.

You will want to convey respect for your patients as well as for your fellow team members by presenting in a professional manner. Thus, you will need to eliminate any foul language or slang terminology from your presentations. You will also want to think about applying general principles of public speaking to your presentations. For example, oral case presentations should be polished and free from extraneous words or phrases such as "uhh" or "you know." Adopting this type of professional presentational style will add to the overall impression you make when presenting your cases.

Success Tip #47
Your presentations should be professional and avoid foul language, slang terminology, and extraneous non-words such as "uhh."

Mistake **#97**

Not including a biopsychosocial formulation

After presenting the details of the case, including the history of present illness, past histories, mental status exam, and relevant diagnostic studies, students may make the mistake of stopping short in their presentation. It is important to be sure to finish your presentation by including a biopsychosocial formulation in which you mention and briefly discuss the significance of biological, psychological, and social factors that influence the presentation and contribute to the diagnostic picture of the particular patient. This approach will allow for a more sophisticated conceptualization of the patient and provide a basis from which to construct more specific and thorough treatment interventions. The biopsychosocial framework for conceptualizing patients is discussed in more detail in Chapter 5.

Success Tip #48

Including a biopsychosocial formulation in your presentation will show that you have an advanced understanding of your patient and of psychiatry, which will certainly advance your grade.

Mistake **#98**

Oversimplifying the diagnostic picture

When presenting your diagnosis, you will want to offer a differential diagnosis, briefly discussing the several most likely diagnoses, particularly if the patient offers a more complicated case or presents a particular diagnostic dilemma. If so, mention this specifically and discuss the most likely diagnoses and provide concise reasons supporting and/or refuting the likelihood of each diagnosis. You should then select a working diagnosis, the most likely diagnosis for the patient at the present time, upon which you will base immediate treatment decisions.

Mistake **#99**

Not giving a multiaxial diagnosis

The multiaxial diagnosis is required for all presentations on your psychiatry clerkship. The diagnoses you list on Axis I and Axis II should be your working diagnoses, upon which you should base your treatment plan. Don't neglect to present Axis III-V. Components of the patient's problems listed here will also need to be addressed in your treatment plan.

Success Tip #49
After discussing your differential diagnosis, give your working diagnoses in the standard multiaxial format.

Mistake **#100**

Not including treatment recommendations in your oral case presentation

For one reason or another, it can be easy for students to consider their task complete when they have presented a case and offered a diagnosis. However, the oral case presentation is incomplete until a treatment plan has been formulated. Your attending or team members may disagree with your treatment plan at times, but your efforts will be applauded.

Mistake **#101**

The treatment plan does not include further investigations that you need to perform

To ensure a thorough treatment plan, you should mention any further information collecting tasks you would like to perform to help clarify the diagnosis. These tasks may include seeking collateral information from family members, previous or current physicians or therapists, and the medical record. You will also want to mention further laboratory studies or diagnostic procedures that you wish to obtain to aid in diagnosis. By convention, these actions are considered to be part of the patient's treatment.

Mistake #102

Not approaching therapeutic interventions from a biopsychosocial perspective

In order for a psychiatric treatment plan to be sufficiently thorough, like the formulation of the case mentioned above, it must address biological, psychological, and social perspectives. You will not want to neglect this concept when you present your cases orally. You should describe appropriately indicated biological, psychological, and social treatments. Again, refer to Chapter 5 for more information on the biopsychosocial treatment plan.

Success Tip #50
Discussing your treatment plan in a biopsychosocial format will help ensure that your plan addresses each aspect of the patient's condition.

Mistake #103

Not seeking feedback on your oral case presentation

You will be doing oral case presentations for years to come, as a student, as a resident, and as a consulting physician, so take this opportunity to improve your skills. Ask your resident and your attending for constructive criticism and use their feedback to improve your performance in future case presentations.

Chapter 7

Commonly Made Mistakes On

Daily Progress Notes

You will likely be expected to write daily progress notes for each of your patients in order to document updates in your patients' care. The notes should give anyone reading the chart a clear idea of each patient's hospital course. All of the pertinent information should be summed up in the daily progress notes, allowing the reader to gather all of this information in one place, rather than flipping incessantly through the chart. Other healthcare providers will read your daily progress notes, especially the assessment and plan, to keep up with what is happening with the patient. There is also a possibility that the patient may eventually read the chart. Finally, remember that the medical record is a legal document. Be sure that your entries would stand up well if the record ends up in court. In this section, we will discuss the common mistakes made in writing daily progress notes.

Mistake **#104**

Underestimating the significance of the daily progress note

You should not make the mistake of underestimating the significance of the daily progress note. Though this exercise may at first appear simple and routine, it is an opportunity for you to shine as a student. The progress note is one of the chief means through which your resident and attending physician will follow *your progress* on the psychiatry rotation. It is important that you express through your notes that you understand key concepts of psychiatric illness and its treatment and that you appreciate the clinical status of your patients. Ideally, as you progress through your rotation, the quality and sophistication of your notes will improve as your knowledge expands and your understanding of psychiatry deepens.

Mistake **#105**

Not writing legibly

Physicians are notorious for bad handwriting, but don't make the mistake of seeking this same notoriety. Your note is worthless if it is illegible, and your grade will reflect it. Others have to be able to read your note for it to be helpful. Even worse, in the hands of a malpractice attorney, an illegible note is a prescription for disaster. It is worth taking the few extra moments to make sure that your handwriting is easily decipherable.

Mistake **#106**

Scribbling out errors

Because the medical record is a legal document, you must not scribble out errors to the point that they are illegible. Instead, cross out the error with a single line and label it "error." Write your initial and the date. To black out a section of the record raises suspicion that you were trying to hide something.

Mistake #107

Placing unnecessary markings in the chart

Your notes should not contain any extraneous markings, such as underlining, stars, etc. Notations such as these may become problematic if the record goes to court. Your notes should be written clearly and concisely, without any unnecessary commentary or markings.

Mistake #108

Bickering with other providers in the chart

Nothing looks worse when a chart is subpoenaed than providers bickering with one another in chart notes. This is not only highly unprofessional, but it also casts enormous doubt upon the quality of care that a patient is receiving. A situation like this may develop when the primary team and a consultant disagree about how a patient should be managed. In general, disagreements between providers should be settled outside of the medical record. The record should document and reflect calm and rational decision-making rather than heated, overly emotional debates.

Success Tip #51

Because the medical record be subpoenaed, care must be exercised when writing notes in the chart. Clinicians must consider how their notes might look if the case ends up in court and be sure that they are not providing ammunition for a malpractice attorney to use against them.

Mistake #109

Omitting the date and time of the note

Each progress note must include the date and time indicating when it was written. This documentation is essential for medical and legal reasons and will assist a reader in following the course of the patient's care when reviewing the chart. Get into the habit of putting the date and time on every entry that you make in the chart.

Mistake #110

Not identifying the type of note you are writing

At the top of your note, next to the date and time, include the title of your note. The title should indicate your level of training as well as the type of note you are writing. Be sure to include your service if you are not part of the primary team, i.e., on a consult service.

Examples:

MS3 Psychiatry Progress Note
MS4 Psychiatry Consult Progress Note

Success Tip #52
Make sure that each note contains the date and time, as well as a title that indicates your level of training and the type of note you are writing.

Mistake #111

Not understanding the appropriate content for the psychiatry daily progress note

Generally, the psychiatry daily progress note should take a form similar to the medical SOAP note, which is traditionally comprised of four main sections: the Subjective and Objective data sections and the Assessment and Plan.

Mistake #112

Being unsure of what to include in the subjective section of the note

The subjective section should contain information elicited from the patient's report to you that day, such as events overnight as described by the patient, how the patient slept, and updates on the relevant symptoms that you are monitoring and treating. Also include in this section reports from nurses, technicians, and therapists that provide further information regarding the patient's status. Newly obtained collateral history from the patient's family or other clinicians can also be included here. Be sure to document the source of the additional information.

Mistake #113

Not knowing what to include in the objective section

The objective section should record more quantitative data such as vital signs, the mental status exam, new laboratory values or the results of new diagnostic studies, and medications the patient is currently taking.

Mistake #114

Failing to include the list of current medications

Though perhaps easily omitted, it is essential that each daily psychiatry progress note contain the list of active medications. The current medication list is of particular importance in the psychiatric progress note, as this list will often contain the most relevant information regarding current treatment interventions. A quick glance at the medication list and the plan over a series of progress notes can help the reader track the patient's history of progress and treatment interventions over time.

Mistake #115

Failing to organize the medication list effectively

In order to be most effective, the medication list should be documented in a consistent and organized fashion. One of the most helpful ways to do this is to list psychiatric medications first, at the top of the list. Below those entries, list each non-psychiatric medication the patient is currently taking. Be sure to include the dosage, route of administration, and schedule for each of the psychiatric medications, though this may not be essential for the non-psychiatric medications. Consistently listing both trade names and generic names for the medications is advised for students as it will aid in your learning of this material. Some practitioners may prefer to have separate lists for psychiatric and non-psychiatric medications.

Mistake **#116**

Forgetting to update the note with recent laboratory studies or results of diagnostic procedures

It is essential that you keep abreast of labs and diagnostic studies that have been ordered and include the results in the progress note as soon as they are available. Obviously, you will want to keep up with this information since this type of data will significantly influence your diagnosis and treatment. Documenting this information in the progress note will be part of this process so that the information will be readily available to other team members, clinicians from other services, and other persons who may be reviewing the chart. Also, including this information promptly in the appropriate place in the objective section of your note will allow you to impress your residents and attending physician with your attention to detail. Should this type of information become available to you later in the day after your note is written, it would be useful to write an addendum to your note including the new information and any associated changes in your assessment and plan.

Mistake #117

Not knowing what to include in the assessment and plan sections

The assessment section should consist of two to three sentences describing the patient's basic identifying information, all relevant medical and psychiatric diagnoses, and a brief description of the patient's progress to date and current clinical status. Your attending may also want you to include a multiaxial diagnosis each day. The plan should be organized as a list of the diagnostic and treatment interventions to be provided for the patient.

Mistake #118

Making statements of assessment outside of the appropriate section

The drawing of conclusions or construction of assessments outside of the formal assessment section is considered improper form. In order to avoid making this common mistake, you might conceptualize the sections in the following manner. The subjective and objective sections are intended strictly for the recording of these two different types of factual data and for nothing else. Any commentary upon the significance or potential significance of this data should be reserved for the assessment section. Though it may be tempting to include this type of material in the data oriented sections for the sake of proximity, you should avoid doing so. Obviously, for more complicated cases, particularly those containing diagnostic dilemmas, the assessment may take on greater length than for more routine cases.

Mistake **#119**

Introducing new data in the body of the assessment

Data must first be presented either in the subjective or objective sections, then its significance addressed in the assessment. To include factual information in the assessment that was not first recorded in one of these two previous sections would represent a mistake in form and potentially confuse the reader as well as cast doubt on the reliability of the information in the progress note.

Mistake **#120**

Neglecting to document a thorough plan

One of the most important aspects of your note will be your plan. The plan is the section that everyone will review, so you will want to convey as much relevant information as possible. When documenting your plan, think of all the things your team is currently providing for your patient as well as what else must be done in order to treat the patient. Obviously, information pertaining to such things as management of medications, use of psychotherapy, and diagnostic studies ordered or considered should be included. Additionally, such interventions as acquiring medical records, speaking with family or other clinicians, consulting other hospital services, and discharge planning are just a few examples of items to include in a thorough plan.

```
┌─────────────────────────────────────────────┐
│              Success Tip #53                  │
│  Progress notes should be written in the SOAP │
│  format. Be sure to write information only in │
│         the appropriate section.              │
└─────────────────────────────────────────────┘
```

Mistake #121

Copying the progress note from the previous day

The progress note should not be a mere copy of the previous day's note with the date changed. Each day's progress note should contain information unique to that day and contain an updated assessment and plan. Copying material from previous days will interfere with other readers' ability to follow your notes and discern which material is actually new from day to day. At institutions with computerized medical records, copying and pasting material from previous notes can be particularly dangerous in this regard. A common mistake seen is the copying of inaccurate data into notes day after day. Once again, imagine what a malpractice attorney could say about the care being delivered when the notes are this inaccurate and sloppy. Further, copying and pasting material from other practitioners' notes is considered to be plagiarism.

```
┌─────────────────────────────────────────────┐
│              Success Tip #54                  │
│  Avoid the temptation to copy and paste notes │
│   in computerized medical records. Doing so   │
│   may seem convenient but often leads to      │
│       inaccuracies in the record.             │
└─────────────────────────────────────────────┘
```

Mistake **#122**

Forgetting to sign your name

This mistake occurs more often than you might expect. In addition to dating and timing every entry in the chart, you must also sign every entry. If your note is more than one page long, be sure to sign each page. Under your signature, print your name, level of training, and pager number legibly. Your resident or attending must then co-sign your note before it is placed in the chart.

Mistake **#123**

Not learning from the resident notes

Residents have become seasoned veterans in the writing of daily progress notes and will have a lot of helpful information to aid you in the development of your note writing skills. They will also likely be able to provide you with information regarding your attending physician's preferences in this arena. You would be well advised to review the residents' notes for pointers that you may incorporate into your note writing. Be sure to also ask your residents for regular feedback on your notes.

Mistake **#124**

Not writing your note early in the day

You should write your notes early in the day, either as part of your pre-rounds or immediately following morning rounds. This will allow ample time for your resident or attending to review and co-sign your note. It will also make the information that you have included in your note available to other clinicians. You shouldn't wait for pending test results to return to complete your note. If you need to add or change something in your note later in the day, you can do so with an addendum.

Success Tip #55

Write your notes early in the day so that they may be reviewed and co-signed by the resident and placed in the chart.

Mistake **#125**

Changing your note after it has been placed in the chart

Once again, the medical record is a legal document that should not be changed or edited once placed in the chart. If you need to change something in your note, start a new note with the date and time and label it "Addendum." You can then add or correct information from the previous note.

Example:

Date/Time
Addendum to MS3 Psychiatry Progress Note
Vital signs in the above note are incorrect. The correct vital signs are...

Success Tip #56

Don't change your note after it has been placed in the chart. Instead, write an addendum to your note, with the current date and time and any necessary additions or corrections.

Mistake **#126**

Not seeking feedback on the quality of your progress notes

As stated above, your progress notes are often a good indicator of your progress on the rotation. Be sure to ask for feedback from your resident and attending on how you might improve your notes. Be proactive in seeking feedback and make the recommended changes a part of your note writing style.

Example of Medical Student Progress Note

Psychiatry Service MS III Note

Date
Time

S: Pt reported complaints, relevant social developments, clinical symptoms you are following including sleep, appetite, mood, anxiety, suicidal/homicidal ideation, hallucinations, delusions, etc. as described by the patient.

O: VS: T   BP   HR   RR

MSE:	*MEDS:*
Gen: 58 y/o WM in hospital attire, well-groomed, appearing his stated age, lying in bed in NAD, reading newspaper	*sertraline 50 mg po qd* *clonazepam 0.5 mg po tid* *trazodone 50 mg po qhs* *propranolol* *isordil*
Sensorium: alert and fully oriented	*albuterol*
Attitude: pleasant and cooperative with interview	*atrovent*

Psychomotor: no significant agitation or retardation
Speech: nl rate/tone/volume
Mood: fine
Affect: full range and congruent
*Thought Content: appropriate, no delusional content, no
paranoia, no SI/HI*
*Thought Processes: logical and goal directed, no
evidence of thought disorder*
Perceptual: no AVH
Insight: good
Judgment: good

LABS: relevant labs (esp. drug levels)
STUDIES: MRI, CT, EEG, EKG, etc.
*A/P: Pt is a 58 y/o WM with major depressive disorder,
PTSD, HTN, CAD, COPD, doing well with stable mood
on sertraline; clonazepam covering anxiety; trazodone
effective for insomnia.*

*1. Continue sertraline 50MG PO QD for depression,
PTSD.*
2. Continue clonazepam 0.5MG PO TID for anxiety.
3. Continue trazodone prn for insomnia.
4. Will provide supportive psychotherapy as needed.

Joe Medstudent, MSIII
Pager Number

Chapter 8

Commonly Made Mistakes During

Team Rounds

During your psychiatry rotation you are likely to round with a multidisciplinary team, especially on an inpatient unit. The members of the team will vary but will generally include an attending psychiatrist, residents, students, nurses, social workers, occupational therapists, and perhaps a chaplain. During team rounds each patient will be discussed with a focus on the patient's progress toward discharge. Each team member will contribute to the treatment plan for each patient. This chapter reviews mistakes commonly made by students during team rounds.

Mistake #127

Not understanding the attending psychiatrist's role

The attending psychiatrist is the leader of the team and is in charge of making sure that the patients assigned to the team are receiving the best care possible. He or she is also responsible for teaching residents and students. The attending will likely see all of the new patients and may or may not see established patients routinely. He or she will guide the treatment plan based upon what is reported about each patient from the various members of the team.

Mistake #128

Not understanding the residents' role

The residents are responsible for the day-to-day care of the patients, along with the attending. Residents make sure that orders are written, studies are performed, and that patients are receiving the care outlined in the treatment plan. As a student, you should strive to perform like a resident. Make sure that you are following up on all orders and studies and that you are spending time with your patients. The more you are involved in the day-to-day care of your patients, the more time the residents will have for their other duty, which is teaching you.

Mistake #129

Overlooking the contributions of psychiatric nurses and technicians

The physicians and students on the team will spend part of their day with the patients, but the nurses and technicians are with the patients every day, evening, and night. They are often able to provide information that residents and students cannot gather or observe. For instance, some patients act very differently whenever someone in a white coat is on the unit. How they behave with other staff members may be a better indicator of how they are actually doing. The nurses on psychiatry units are responsible for carrying out the orders of the physicians. They may also provide therapy for patients as needed and often have additional information that the patient has shared with them. The psychiatric technicians work closely with the nursing staff by helping to make

sure that the unit is safe for patients and staff. They also
spend time with the patients, playing games or
conducting groups.

Mistake **#130**

Not understanding the role of the social workers

Social workers try to help patients with a wide array of
needs, such as discharge planning, housing, disability
paperwork, commitment paperwork, and so forth. Many
social workers also have advanced clinical training and
perform individual and group psychotherapy with
patients. The social worker assigned to a patient may
also be involved in family meetings, along with the
resident and student caring for the patient.

Mistake **#131**

Overlooking the contribution of occupational therapists on the unit

The occupational therapists help patients with grooming
and hygiene, as well as leading activity groups, such as
music, games, crafts, cooking, etc. They may also
organize outings to movies, parks, etc. They will be able
to provide important information regarding whether the
patient is able to care for himself or not, which will help
determine readiness for discharge.

Success Tip #57

Each member of the team is important to the overall care of the patients. Be sure that you understand and appreciate the valuable contributions made by each team member.

Mistake **#132**

Not sharing information with the team

Confidentiality dictates that information must be kept within the team, but all clinical information should be shared with all team members. If your patient asks you to withhold information from the team, explain that all of the team members are trying to help him and that in order to do their job, the team needs to know what is going on with him. Being very open and frank during team rounds helps minimize splitting by patients, which, if uncontrolled, can wreak havoc on a unit.

Success Tip #58

All information gathered should be shared with the team. Open communication within the team helps minimize splitting off of team members.

Mistake **#133**

Not being prepared to interview patients during team rounds

Often during team rounds, new patients are interviewed by the resident or student in front of the team. You will generally be able to observe the resident or attending interview before you are expected to do so. The team interview is beneficial to the patient by reducing the repetition of numerous interviews. As reviewed in mistake #20, it is important to try to make the patient feel at ease in the group interview. By making the patient feel comfortable, you will show the attending that you are able to make an empathic connection with the patient.

Mistake #134

Not interviewing concisely during team rounds

Be sure that you ask how much time you have to interview the patient during rounds. You should generally take about 15-20 minutes to gather a history and perform the mental status exam and mini-mental status exam, if indicated. If a patient is especially long-winded or tangential, you will need to redirect him. Here is another opportunity to impress your attending with your skills. Try to leave a couple of minutes at the end for other team members to ask questions as well.

Mistake #135

Trying to cover everything in a team interview

You should not try to get every detail of the patient's life history during the team interview. Focus on the HPI and past psychiatric history, including substance use, and then use the remaining time to ask about medical history, social, and developmental history. You can always go back and fill in the gaps after rounds.

Success Tip #59

Interviews conducted during team rounds should be focused and take no more than 15 to 20 minutes. Use this as an opportunity to show off your interviewing skills to your attending.

Chapter 9

Commonly Made Mistakes During

The Oral Examination

In addition to a written examination, many medical schools include an oral examination in the overall evaluation of students' performances on the psychiatry clerkship. It is usually one of the more anxiously anticipated parts of the clerkship, though adequate preparation and practice can help you perform well. Even if your school does not conduct oral exams, the tips included here will be useful for any presentation. Mistakes commonly made by students during the oral examination are discussed in this chapter.

Mistake **#136**

Not learning about the exam in advance

You will want to find out early in the rotation whether you have an oral exam and how the exam is structured. Oral exams may include an interview of a live or standardized patient, viewing a videotaped interview and then presenting the case, and/or case vignettes that you will be expected to discuss. The clerkship director should be able to provide information about the exam, but medical students who have already completed the clerkship and your residents will also be good sources of information.

Mistake #137

Not practicing interviewing patients

During your clerkship, you should interview a large number of patients with different diagnoses. Hopefully, some of these interviews will be observed by your resident and attending. Interviewing a patient while being observed is more difficult than interviewing alone, so make sure that you get plenty of practice interviewing with someone watching. Be sure to ask your resident or attending to give you feedback on your interview style.

Mistake #138

Not practicing oral presentations

You should have ample opportunity to practice presenting patients during your rotation. If not, ask your resident or attending to listen to you present the patients you evaluate. Practicing the order in which you need to present and learning to stay within a 10-15 minute time frame will help you prepare for your oral exam. Also, the more oral presentations you give, the more comfortable you will be presenting in front of someone.

Success Tip #60
The best way to alleviate anxiety about the oral exam is to find out about the exam beforehand and practice, practice, practice.

Mistake #139

Being unsure about what information to collect and present

The oral examination patient interview and/or presentation will be similar to those that you did on your rotation. You should be thorough and include the following information:

- Chief complaint

- History of present illness

- Review of psychiatric symptoms

- Past psychiatric history

- Past medical and surgical history

- Medications

- Medication allergies

- Family history (especially family psychiatric history)

- Social and developmental history

- Mental status exam

- Biopsychosocial formulation

- Differential diagnosis

- DSM-IV multiaxial diagnoses

- Biopsychosocial treatment plan

Mistake #140

Omitting information not covered in the videotaped interview

If you are watching a videotaped interview of a patient, a complete history may not be obtained. However, during your presentation you will still want to mention each component of the history and mental status exam. If the interviewer did not elicit the information, you should say that it was not covered in the interview. In your plan, you can say that you would go back and clarify those areas. This shows your examiner that you know what information needs to be gathered in a psychiatric evaluation.

Success Tip #61

In your presentation, point out any information that was not obtained in the interview and state in your plan that you would gather further history.

Mistake #141

Not discussing suicidality thoroughly

In addition to testing your fund of knowledge of psychiatry, the oral exam is aimed at determining whether you can practice safely when caring for patients with psychiatric illness. Even if you do not specialize in psychiatry, you will be seeing patients with psychiatric illness. You will be responsible for determining whether they need to be referred to see a psychiatrist or hospitalized for safety. The most important aspect of evaluating patient safety is a thorough assessment of suicidality. Therefore, be sure that you adequately discuss suicidality in your case presentation. You need to talk about the patient's admission or denial of suicidal thoughts, plan, and intent, as well as suicide risk factors. Be sure to include hospitalization in your treatment plan if suicidality is present. If someone else interviews the patient and does not ask about suicidality, be sure to mention that suicidality was not covered and that you would go back and ask the patient about this.

Mistake **#142**

Not mentioning homicidal thoughts or plans

Like suicidality, homicidality must be covered in your presentation. Even if the interviewer did not ask about homicidality specifically, mention it in your presentation so that your examiners know that you thought about this important safety issue.

Success Tip #62
A thorough discussion of suicidality and homicidality is imperative to convince your examiners that you can safely assess patients.

Mistake **#143**

Neglecting to adequately discuss substance use

Because substance use can mimic so many psychiatric symptoms, it is an important part of every patient evaluation. Be sure to discuss the patient's substance use, including pointing out important pieces of information that may not have been elicited.

Success Tip #63
Substance use should be assessed with every patient and discussed in every presentation.

Mistake #144

Not developing a thorough differential diagnosis

By developing and presenting a thorough differential diagnosis, you can show that you know the diagnostic criteria for major psychiatric illnesses. You should mention all of the possible diagnoses and then discuss the evidence that supports and/or refutes each diagnosis. Be sure that you know diagnostic criteria, including the time criteria, for illnesses such as Major Depressive Disorder, Bipolar Disorder, and Schizophrenia (reviewed in Appendix C).

Mistake #145

Forgetting to mention substance use and general medical conditions in your differential diagnosis

Remember that substance intoxication and withdrawal and many general medical conditions can mimic or exacerbate psychiatric symptoms. Therefore, your

differential diagnosis should always include illnesses
secondary to substances or general medical conditions.
You may state that the likelihood of such conditions is
low, but be sure that you mention the possibility in your
discussion.

Success Tip #64
A thorough differential diagnosis must include
illnesses secondary to substance use and general
medical conditions.

Mistake #146

Omitting the multiaxial diagnosis

After discussing your differential diagnosis, present your
working diagnoses using the multiaxial format. Though
you will not likely give a personality disorder diagnosis
based upon one interview, don't simply "defer" an Axis II
diagnosis. Discuss personality traits suggested by the
interview that might contribute to a personality disorder.
Remember to include medical conditions on Axis III,
stressors on Axis IV, and the Global Assessment of
Functioning on Axis V (calculating the GAF is explained
in Appendix G).

Success Tip #65
Be sure to include a multiaxial diagnosis in your
presentation. Familiarize yourself with what
information goes on each axis.

113

Mistake #147

Not following a biopsychosocial approach for the formulation and treatment plan

As with all of your presentations, you will impress your examiners by giving a biopsychosocial formulation for the case. Once again, doing so will help you tie together the various aspects of the patient's life that may be contributing to his or her illness. Following this approach for your treatment plan will also ensure that you include each of the necessary aspects of treatment. The biopsychosocial formulation and treatment plan are detailed further in Chapter 5.

Mistake #148

Not knowing how to manage medications from each of the major classes of psychotropics

In the biological section of your treatment plan, you will likely be expected to discuss medications that you would use to treat the patient. You will need to choose a medication to treat the patient and support your choice with clinical information specific to the patient. You will also need to discuss the evaluation you would conduct, such as laboratory tests or studies that you would order, before starting this particular medication. You will then discuss the dosing of the medication, possible side effects, adverse effects, and any required laboratory monitoring.

For each major category of psychiatric illness, know at least a couple of medications from the appropriate class well enough to discuss them in detail. Your examiner will likely quiz you on the above information if you do not offer it in your treatment plan. Review Appendix D to learn the information that you must know about commonly used psychotropic medications.

Success Tip #66
Know several medications for each illness well enough to discuss them in detail.

Mistake **#149**

Failing to include psychological and social treatments in your plan

Most patients would benefit from some sort of psychotherapy, ranging from insight-oriented psychotherapy to supportive and educational therapies. Be sure that you consider psychotherapy and include it in your treatment plan, in addition to medications. If the patient's family is involved, consider family therapy or family education. Family interventions, along with community services such as housing and financial support, will address the social aspects of the patient's care. Neglecting these important parts of the treatment plan will likely result in a lower grade.

Success Tip #67
A complete treatment plan must include any psychotherapy and social services necessary to adequately treat the patient.

Mistake #150

Appearing unprofessional

The issue of professionalism makes a fitting conclusion to this book, as professionalism is important in every aspect of medical practice. In all situations, from encounters with patients, to interactions with members of the team, to oral case presentations, you should always look and act professionally. In your oral examination, in particular, be sure that you are dressed neatly and appropriately. As discussed in previous sections, avoid using foul language or slang terminology. Try to minimize the use of non-words and extraneous phrases such as "uhh," "like," or "you know." Practicing your presentations, either with an audience or alone, will help you feel more comfortable and become more polished. You will certainly impress your examiners with a professional appearance and confident presentation.

Success Tip #68

Professionalism includes maintaining an appropriate appearance and strong work ethic, working well with colleagues, and taking responsibility for your patients' care. It is never too early in your medical career to be professional.

Appendix A

Ward Etiquette

Certain unwritten rules are essential for your success on the psychiatry rotation. Many of these are consistent with your other rotations, although there are some that are specific to psychiatry.

- **Never use the word "crazy" when describing a patient.** This and other disparaging terms may be offensive to patients, their families, staff, residents and attendings

- **Always be on time.** Never have the team wait for you.

- **Be enthusiastic and attentive at all times.**

- **When you complete your work, help others with theirs.** Everyone likes a team player.

- **Dress professionally.** Studies show that physicians who dress professionally have better relations with their patients, and their patients tend to be more compliant.

- **If you don't know, admit it.** It's best to say you don't know but will find out.

- **Don't scoop your classmates or resident.** Being a team player means not showing up team members.

- **Remember to date and time every entry in the chart.**

- **Make sure that you get all of your notes co-signed.** This ensures that your resident knows that you are following your patients closely and streamlines work for them.

- **If your patient is not doing well, notify your team immediately.**

- **Respect patient confidentiality.** Never talk about a patient in a public place, even if you don't initiate the conversation. Also, make sure that you keep all patient records in a secure place and that they are properly disposed of when they are no longer needed.

- **Be as efficient as possible, and practice at increasing efficiency every day.** The sooner you learn to be efficient, the better.

- **Never leave without permission.** Always check out with your resident before you leave. Ask if there is anything that you can do for them before you go.

- **Strive to be "careful, quick, and kind."** To sum up…be careful to be thorough and conscientious, be quick in getting your work done, and be kind to patients, their families, team members and staff. This is a never-fail recipe for success.

Appendix B

Tips (General Pearls)

Here are some general tips that will help you be a success in your clerkship.

- Before the rotation starts, ask other students who have completed the rotation for some tips and advice. Find out what resources others have found useful for the rotation. Knowing what to study can make a huge difference on the exam.

- Familiarize yourself with the setting. Know where to find computers, charts, forms, and medication administration records in the nursing unit. Learn where the bathrooms are located.

- Make sure that you are prepared with all the right tools for the rotation. In psychiatry, this means that you know how to perform a mental status examination, including cognitive testing, and a neurological examination.

- Review how to read head CTs and MRIs before the rotation. If you are knowledgeable about these studies, you will definitely impress your resident and attending.

- Keep a little notebook and pen with you at all times to write down important bits of information mentioned throughout the rotation. Much of this information will come up on your written or oral exams.

- Whenever you give talks to the team, make handouts that are short, direct, and useful.

- Check your patient's medication list daily. This will help ensure that all of the team members are clear on which medications your patient is receiving.

- See your patients at least twice a day. By spending more time with patients in the afternoon, morning prerounds will go much faster.

- Read about all of the patients assigned to the team, not just your own. You may be asked questions about any patient, so be prepared.

- If you have an oral examination at the end of your rotation, use every patient presentation as an opportunity to practice. The more comfortable you are giving presentations, the better you will do on your exam.

Appendix C
"Must Know" Reviews

A number of disorders you can be assured you will see and be tested on during your psychiatry clerkship. This review, while not exhaustive, contains information that you must know to succeed on your rotation and your exam.

Major Depressive Disorder

Five or more of the following for two weeks; at least one must be depressed mood or loss of interest or pleasure:
- Depressed mood most of the day, nearly every day
- Loss of interest or pleasure in most activities, most of the day
- Change in appetite
- Insomnia/hypersomnia nearly every day
- Psychomotor agitation/retardation
- Decreased energy
- Feelings of worthlessness/guilt
- Decreased concentration
- Suicidal

Symptoms cause significant distress or impairment in social, occupational, or other important areas of functioning.

Symptoms do not meet criteria for mixed episode, are not due to the direct physiological effects of a substance or general medical condition, and are not better accounted for by bereavement.

Specifiers: mild, moderate, severe, chronic, psychotic features, catatonic features, melancholic features, atypical features, postpartum onset, seasonal pattern.

Characteristic	Description
Melancholic Features	Severe anhedonia (loss of all interest/pleasure), early morning awakening, weight loss, profound feelings of guilt; also called "endogenous depression" because of lack of external precipitants
Atypical Features	Overeating and oversleeping; more likely to respond to monoamine oxidase inhibitors (MAOIs)
Psychotic Features	Occur only in presence of mood symptoms (otherwise consider diagnosis of schizoaffective disorder); responds especially well to ECT
Lifetime Prevalence	10-25% for women; 5-12% for men
Mean Age of Onset	40 years
Genetic Link	First-degree relatives of persons with MDD are 2-3 times more likely to have MDD than normal controls
Recurrence	After first episode, 50% chance of relapse; after second episode, 60-70% chance of relapse; after third episode, >90% chance of relapse (will likely need lifelong treatment)
Duration	6 to 13 months untreated; about 3 months treated
Course of Illness	Over time, episodes occur more frequently, last longer, and are more severe
Suicidality	Approximately one-third of depressed people contemplate suicide; 10-15% commit suicide

Characteristic	Description
Bipolar Disorder	5 to 10% of those initially diagnosed with MDD will have a manic episode within 10 years
Anxiety	90% of depressed patients report anxiety and many have a comorbid anxiety disorder
Beck's Cognitive Triad	(1) negative views about the self, (2) tendency to experience the world as hostile and demanding, and (3) expectation of a future filled with suffering and failure

Bipolar Disorder

Manic Episode

Persistently elevated, expansive, or irritable mood, lasting at least one week (or any duration if hospitalization is necessary), plus three of the following (four if mood is only irritable):

- Inflated self-esteem or grandiosity
- Decreased need for sleep
- More talkative than usual or pressure to keep talking
- Flight of ideas, or experience that thoughts are racing
- Easily distracted
- Increased goal directed activity (work, social, sex) or psychomotor agitation
- Excessive involvement in pleasurable activities that have a high potential for painful consequences (shopping sprees, hypersexuality, foolish business investments)

Symptoms cause significant distress or impairment in social, occupational, or other important areas of functioning, or necessitate hospitalization, or include psychotic features

Symptoms do not meet criteria for mixed episode, are not due to the direct physiological effects of a substance (including antidepressant treatment) or general medical condition

Hypomanic Episode

Symptoms last at least four days, and disturbances in mood and change in functioning are observable by others but are not severe enough to cause marked impairment in functioning or to necessitate hospitalization, and there are no psychotic features.

Mixed Episode

Criteria are met for both a manic episode and a major depressive episode (except for duration) nearly every day for at least one week and mood disturbance is severe enough to cause significant distress or impairment in social, occupational, or other important areas of functioning, or necessitate hospitalization, or include psychotic features.

Characteristic	Description
Bipolar I Disorder	Must have had at least one manic episode
Bipolar II Disorder	Must have had at least one hypomanic episode and one major depressive episode and never have had a manic or mixed episode

Characteristic	Description
Rapid Cycling	Specifier for bipolar I or II disorder that requires at least four episodes of mood disturbance in the previous twelve months; occurs in 5-15% of persons with bipolar disorder
Lifetime Prevalence	1-2% for men and women
Peak Age of Onset	16-24 years
Genetic Link	First-degree relatives of persons with bipolar I disorder are 8-18 times more likely to have bipolar I disorder and 2-10 times more likely to have MDD than normal controls; 50% of persons with bipolar I disorder have at least one parent with a mood disorder
Recurrence	>90% (requires lifelong treatment)
Duration	19 weeks for depressive episodes, 10 weeks for manic episodes, 36 weeks for mixed episodes
Course of Illness	Begins as depression in 75% of women and 67% of men; as illness progresses, time between episodes decreases
Prognosis	Worse than MDD; one-third of patients with bipolar I disorder have chronic symptoms and evidence of significant social decline
Suicidality	10-15% commit suicide (may occur in any mood state)
Good Prognosticators	Short duration of manic episodes, advanced age of onset, few suicidal ideations, few comorbid psychiatric or medical problems

Characteristic	Description
Poor Prognosticators	Premorbid poor occupational status, substance abuse disorder, psychotic features, depressive features, inter-episode depressive features, male gender

Schizophrenia

Two or more of the following for a significant portion of time during a 1 month period (or only one if delusions are bizarre or hallucinations consist of a voice keeping up a running commentary on the person's behavior or thoughts, or two or more voices conversing with one another):

- Delusions
- Hallucinations
- Disorganized speech (frequent derailment or incoherence)
- Grossly disorganized or catatonic behavior
- Negative symptoms (affective flattening, alogia or avolition)

Symptoms cause significant distress or impairment in social, occupational, or other important areas of functioning.

Continuous signs of the disturbance persist for at least 6 months with at least 1 month of symptoms.

Symptoms do not meet criteria for schizoaffective disorder or mood disorder with psychotic features and are not due to the direct physiological effects of a substance or general medical condition.

Subtypes

- **Paranoid type.** Preoccupation with delusions or frequent auditory hallucinations; disorganized speech/behavior and flat affect are not prominent.

- **Disorganized type.** Disorganized speech and behavior and flat or inappropriate affect are all prominent.

- **Catatonic type.** At least of two of the following: motoric immobility (catalepsy, waxy flexibility, stupor), excessive purposeless motor activity, extreme negativism or mutism, peculiar voluntary movement (posturing, stereotypies, grimacing).

- **Undifferentiated type.** None of above criteria are met.

- **Residual type.** Absence of prominent positive symptoms; continued presence of negative symptoms and attenuated positive symptoms.

Schizoaffective Disorder

Criteria for mood disorder (MDD, manic or mixed episode) and schizophrenia are met within an uninterrupted period of illness; during same illness, there have been delusions and hallucinations for at least 2 weeks in the absence of mood symptoms.

Characteristic	Description
Positive Symptoms	Delusions and hallucinations
Negative Symptoms	Affective flattening, poverty of speech or speech content, blocking, poor grooming, lack of motivation, anhedonia, social withdrawal
Lifetime Prevalence	1% in men and women

Characteristic	Description
Peak Age of Onset	10-25 years for men; 25-35 years for women
Seasonal Link	Persons with schizophrenia are more likely to have been born in winter and early spring (January to April in Northern Hemisphere and July to September in Southern Hemisphere)
Genetic Link	First-degree relatives with 10-fold increased risk when compared with normal controls; monozygotic twin concordance of 47%
Course of Illness	Exacerbations and remissions with stepwise deterioration in baseline functioning following each relapse; positive symptoms may become less severe with time but negative symptoms increase and are socially debilitating
Prognosis	Poorer than mood disorders; 20-30% may lead somewhat normal lives; 20-30% continue to experience moderate symptoms; 40-60% remain significantly impaired for life
Suicidality	15% commit suicide
Good Prognosticators	Positive symptoms, late onset, obvious precipitating factors, acute onset, good premorbid functioning, mood disorder symptoms, family history of mood disorders, good support systems, married, paranoid type

Characteristic	Description
Poor Prognosticators	Negative symptoms, young onset, insidious onset with no precipitants, poor premorbid functioning, withdrawn or autistic behavior, single, family history of schizophrenia, poor support systems, neurological signs/ symptoms, history of perinatal trauma, no remissions in 3 years, many relapses, history of assaultiveness
Bleuler's Fundamental (Primary) Symptoms	Associations (loose), Affect (blunted), Autism, Ambivalence
Downward Drift Hypothesis	Persons with schizophrenia tend to move into, or fail to rise out of, a low socioeconomic group
Eye Movement Dysfunction	Traits of schizophrenia include disorders of smooth visual pursuit and disinhibition of saccadic eye movements

Personality Disorders

Personality disorders are defined as **pervasive, persistent, and maladaptive** patterns of behavior that are **long-standing and deeply ingrained.** This pattern may be apparent in how a person perceives and interprets himself and the world, in affectivity, in interpersonal functioning, and in impulse control. The personality disorders are divided into three clusters. Each personality disorder has diagnostic criteria, but it is generally more helpful for students to learn to recognize patterns of behavior suggestive of a personality disorder than to memorize a DSM-IV list. Many patients will **exhibit traits of more than one personality disorder,** and there is significant overlap in the symptoms of the personality disorders. Because personality disorders are usually diagnosed after establishing a history with a patient and observing their behavior over time, you will likely use a "rule-out ___ personality disorder" diagnosis in your patient encounters and oral exam during your clerkship. Moreover, most patients with personality disorders will **also have an Axis I disorder.** Remember, too, that when a patient is stressed, i.e. in the throes of a major depressive episode, personality features may be exaggerated. Therefore, personality disorders should ideally be diagnosed when a patient is euthymic.

You should also keep in mind that you will see patients with personality disorders in every patient care specialty, so use your psychiatry clerkship to better understand these patients. This will enable you to care for them in a more compassionate and tolerant way in the future. A good rule of thumb is to remind yourself that a severe personality disorder can be just as debilitating as MDD or bipolar disorder, causing the patient long-term difficulties in life. These patients have often had terrible childhoods that have contributed to their maladaptive way of dealing with the world. Further, they generally don't "choose" to utilize poor coping skills; it comes as "second nature." By understanding some of these basic premises, you will probably find it a little easier to empathize with these patients.

Cluster A. "Odd and Eccentric"

- **Paranoid Personality Disorder.** Characterized by **long-standing suspiciousness** and **mistrust of others.** They can't accept their own feelings and thoughts, instead assigning them to others. This defense mechanism is called **projection.** The best approach to dealing with these patients is to be non-defensive and straightforward. You shouldn't agree with their injustice collecting, but should avoid challenging it.

● **Schizoid Personality Disorder.** Characterized by *social withdrawal* and *isolation* without the need for close human contact. They often have interest in solitary activities and succeed at lonely jobs that others would find undesirable (e.g., the movie theater projectionist). Importantly, their *reality testing is intact.*

● **Schizotypal Personality Disorder.** Characterized by *strikingly odd or strange behavior, thoughts, affect, speech and appearance.* Although frank thought disorder is absent, these patients often believe that they have special abilities or powers and may have vivid fantasy lives. They generally have few friends and don't really want close human relationships. Schizotypal personality disorder may be a *precursor to schizophrenia,* though this is not the course for everyone with this disorder.

Cluster B. "Dramatic, Emotional, and Erratic"

● **Antisocial Personality Disorder.** Characterized by an *inability to conform to societal norms* and *disregard for the rights of others.* These patients are often quite charming and ingratiating and are able to "con" even the most experienced clinician. These patients will have exhibited symptoms of conduct disorder in childhood. They *lack remorse* for their actions, appearing to lack a conscience. Though these patients generally do not feel anxious or depressed, the presence of these symptoms improves their prognosis. In other words, only people with a conscience get anxious or depressed, so these symptoms signify that they have at least some conscience with which an experienced clinician can work.

- **Borderline Personality Disorder.** Characterized by *impulsivity and instability in many facets of life, including affect, relationships, self-image, and behavior.* Though they push people away with their behavior, they desperately *fear abandonment.* They often make *suicidal threats or attempts.* They mutilate themselves, which helps them feel "real" and "alive," temporarily relieving their intrapsychic pain. The term borderline refers to those patients that stand on the border of neurosis and psychosis. These are some of the most challenging patients to treat, and even the most patient physician can become very frustrated with this type of patient who may unconsciously thwart every effort to help them.

  Once again, remember that these patients have often been victimized in childhood. The only way that they know how to relate to others is as victim or aggressor. They will often leave others feeling victimized. They may also project their aggression onto someone else, which results in the patient being victimized by that person. This defense mechanism is called *projective identification.* For example, the patient may project an intolerable feeling or part of herself, like anger, onto the clinician. The patient then induces the clinician to play the projected role, often by behaving in ways that will result in the clinician becoming angry. The clinician, identifying with the projected feeling of anger, will then act in ways that confirm what has been projected. You might find yourself in the role of a victimizer and say things that you wish you hadn't said. If you find yourself feeling or behaving with a borderline patient in a way that is unlike your usual way of dealing with patients, consider that you and your patient may be engaged in projective identification.

Patients with borderline personality disorder also use *splitting* as a defense mechanism. This is an unconscious division of feelings into all good or all bad. For instance, on the inpatient unit, the patient may idealize some team members and uniformly disparage others, rather than recognizing that everyone has some good qualities and some bad qualities. Listen for phrases like "you're the only person who has ever really listened to me" or "no one understands me but you" that will indicate that you (or another team member) are being idealized. Likewise, listen for "you're the worst doctor (nurse, student, etc.) that I've ever seen" or "you don't understand me the way (the idealized staff member) does." It is important that the team members stay in close communication when treating a borderline patient, as they can split an entire hospital ward, creating chaos for patients and staff alike.

Most students find patients with borderline personality disorder the most challenging patients to treat. Be open and honest about your feelings with your attending and resident, and they can help you find ways to deal with these patients in an effective way.

- **Histrionic Personality Disorder.** Characterized by *dramatic, flamboyant, emotional, and seductive behavior* and a global, impressionistic cognitive style. These patients are *attention seeking* and very needy. They may display temper tantrums if they are not the center of attention. Their *relationships are superficial,* and they lack the ability to build and maintain lasting, meaningful attachments. Unlike borderline patients, those with histrionic personality disorder usually do not attempt suicide and lack the identity diffusion and brief psychotic episodes characteristic in borderline personality disorder. Psychotherapy is aimed at helping these patients identify their inner feelings, of which they are often unaware.

- **Narcissistic Personality Disorder.** Characterized by a *heightened sense of self-importance and grandiosity.* These patients consider themselves special and feel entitled to special treatment by only "the best doctor." They become enraged whenever someone criticizes them (i.e., narcissistic rage). They *lack empathy,* finding it very difficult to identify with anyone else's feelings. Ironically, these patients have very *fragile self-esteems* and are prone to depression whenever their self-esteem is bruised (so-called narcissistic injury). Psychotherapy is aimed at empathic listening and "mirroring." *Mirroring* refers to the clinician reflecting the patient's feelings back to him, like a mother does for a toddler. For instance, whenever the toddler does a dance, the attentive and empathic mother will clap and make a fuss over the child. This empathic connection in the therapy enables the patient to begin to form an authentic and empathic relationship with the therapist, though this takes many years to develop. On your clerkship rotation, you should practice being empathic with these patients.

Cluster C. "Anxious or Fearful"

- **Avoidant Personality Disorder.** Characterized by *extreme sensitivity to rejection.* They are shy and timid and often live socially withdrawn lives. Unlike the schizoid personality, though, these patients *desperately want companionship,* but need unusually high assurance of acceptance. They are often uncertain and self-effacing, lacking self-confidence. Their avoidance of social situations may be *virtually indistinguishable from social anxiety disorder on Axis I.* They may also become depressed or anxious when their limited social support system fails.

● **Dependent Personality Disorder.** Characterized by *submissive and dependent behavior* and *reliance on others* to assume responsibility for their lives and make the majority of their decisions. They may experience **intense discomfort when they are alone** and urgently seek to replace a relationship that has ended. These patients may stay in an abusive relationship to avoid having to make the decision to end the relationship and risk being alone.

● **Obsessive-Compulsive Personality Disorder.** Characterized by *inflexibility and emotional constriction.* These patients are *perfectionistic and indecisive,* characteristics that often lead to difficulty completing projects for fear tdhat they are not yet "perfect." They are *preoccupied with rules, orderliness and neatness.* They have limited interpersonal skills and are often seen as being too serious and lacking a sense of humor. While most successful physicians possess some of these characteristics, patients with OCPD generally are not able to function at this level, which requires flexibility and quick decision-making. OCPD is also distinguished from obsessive-compulsive disorder, an Axis I anxiety disorder that is characterized by obsessions and rituals that cause distress to the patient.

Appendix D: Commonly Used Psychotropic Medications

Table 1. Key Features of Antidepressants

Medication	Usual Daily Dosing Range (mg)	Proposed Mechanism of Action	Side Effects	Other Key Features or Adverse Effects
Tricyclics *Tertiary amine tricyclics* Amitriptyline (Elavil) Clomipramine (Anafranil) Doxepin (Sinequan) Imipramine (Tofranil) *Secondary amine tricyclics* Desipramine (Norpramin) Nortriptyline (Pamelor)	100-300 100-250 100-300 100-300 100-300 50-150	5-HT + NE reuptake inhibition	Anticholinergic effects[1], orthostasis, sedation, weight gain, sexual dysfunction	Lethal in overdose; quinidine-like effects on cardiac conduction; lower seizure threshold
Selective Serotonin Reuptake Inhibitors Citalopram (Celexa) Escitalopram (Lexapro) Fluoxetine (Prozac, Serafem) Fluvoxamine (Luvox) Paroxetine (Paxil, Paxil CR) Sertraline (Zoloft)	20-60 10-20 20-60 50-300 20-60 50-200	5-HT reuptake inhibition	Initial: nausea, diarrhea, headache, insomnia, agitation/anxiety Ongoing: sexual dysfunction	Non-lethal in overdose; recent FDA investigation into link between SSRIs and increased risk of suicide resulting in "black box" warning for use in children and adolescents
Bupropion (Wellbutrin SR, XL)	150-400	DA + NE reuptake inhibition	Initial: nausea, headache, insomnia, agitation/anxiety	Lower seizure threshold (esp with comorbid eating disorders)
Venlafaxine (Effexor XR)	75-300	5-HT + NE (+ DA) reuptake inhibition	Same as SSRIs	Hypertension at higher doses

Medication	Dosing Range (mg)	Mechanism of Action	Side Effects	Other Key Features or Adverse Effects
Duloxetine (Cymbalta)	30-60	5-HT + NE reuptake inhibition	Same as SSRIs	Also useful for diabetic neuropathy and stress urinary incontinence
Nefazodone (Serzone)	150-300	5-HT$_2$ receptor antagonism + weak 5-HT + NE reuptake inhibition	Initial: nausea, dizziness, confusion, visual changes, sedation	"Black box" warning for liver failure; no sexual dysfunction
Trazodone (Desyrel)	75-300	5-HT$_2$ receptor antagonism + weak 5-HT reuptake inhibition	Sedation, dizziness, orthostasis	Priapism; cardiac arrhythmias
Mirtazapine (Remeron)	15-45	a_2-Adrenergic + 5-HT$_2$ receptor antagonism	Anticholinergic effects [1], sedation, weight gain, rare orthostasis	May increase serum lipid levels; rare hypertension, peripheral edema, agranulocytosis; no sexual dysfunction
Monoamine Oxidase Inhibitors Phenelzine (Nardil) Tranylcypromine (Parnate)	15-90 30-60	MAO inhibition	Orthostatic hypotension, headache, insomnia, weight gain, sexual dysfunction	Hypertensive crisis (requires dietary restriction of tyramine); potentially life-threatening drug-drug interactions (serotonin syndrome when used with meperidine, antidepressants, sympathomimetics, others); peripheral edema; avoid in pts with CHF; avoid phenelzine in patients with hepatic impairment

5-HT=serotonin; 5-HT$_2$=serotonin type 2 receptor; NE=norepinephrine; DA=dopamine; SSRI=selective serotonin reuptake inhibitor; FDA=U.S. Food and Drug Administration; MAO=monoamine oxidase; CHF=congestive heart failure
1. Anticholinergic side effects include dry mouth, blurred vision, constipation, urinary retention, tachycardia, and confusion.

Table 2. Key Features of Mood Stabilizers[1]

Medication	Usual Daily Dosing Range or Target Blood Level	Required Laboratory Monitoring	Side Effects	Other Key Features or Adverse Effects
Lithium	600-1200 mg 0.8-1.2 mEq/L	Pretreatment: BUN, Cr, electrolytes, CBC, TSH, pregnancy test, ECG (age 40 or older or history of cardiac disease) Ongoing: BUN, Cr, TSH, lithium level every 6-12 months	Fine resting tremor, sedation, weight gain, acne, nausea, diarrhea	Contraindicated in pts with sick sinus syndrome and unstable renal function; risk of Ebstein's anomaly in infants exposed *in utero* (0.1%-0.7%); ECG changes (flattening of T waves); leukocytosis (benign); hypothyroidism (usually reversible); nephrogenic diabetes insipidus (usually reversible); toxicity potentiated by thiazide diuretics; shown in clinical trials to reduce incidence of suicide; adjunct to antidepressants in MDD Toxicity: *Mild* (1.5-2.0 mEq/L): GI upset, coarse tremor, ataxia, dizziness, slurred speech, nystagmus *Moderate* (2.1-2.5 mEq/L): nausea/vomiting, blurred vision, clonus, seizures, delirium, coma, circulatory failure *Severe* (>2.5 mEq/L): generalized seizures, renal failure, death
Valproate (Depakote, Depakote ER, Depakene)	20 mg/kg for rapid stabilization 50-150 mcg/mL	Pretreatment: LFTs, CBC, pregnancy test Ongoing: LFTs, CBC, VPA level every 12 months	Essential tremor, nausea, sedation, weight gain, alopecia	Hepatic toxicity; thrombocytopenia; rare pancreatitis; risk of neural tube defects and craniofacial defects in infants exposed *in utero*; may inhibit hepatic enzymes and raise serum concentrations of phenobarbital, ethosuximide, active 10, 11-epoxide metabolite of carbamazepine, lamotrigine; superior to lithium in patients with rapid-cycling and mixed episodes

Medication	Usual Daily Dosing Range or Target Blood Level	Required Laboratory Monitoring	Side Effects	Other Key Features or Adverse Effects
Carbamazepine (Tegretol, Carbatrol)	400-1200 mg 8-12 mcg/mL (Toxicity may occur even with therapeutic serum level due to elevated levels of the active metabolite, 10,11-epoxide)	Pretreatment: LFTs, CBC, pregnancy test Ongoing: LFTs, CBC, CBZ level every 12 months	Rash, nausea, dizziness, ataxia, sedation	Hepatic toxicity; cholestasis; SIADH (with resultant hyponatremia); agranulocytosis; aplastic anemia; leucopenia; risk of neural tube defects, microcephaly, craniofacial defects in infants exposed in utero; induces hepatic enzymes and reduces levels of oral contraceptives, VPA, self
Oxcarbazepine (Trileptal)	900-2400 mg	Ongoing: Sodium	Dizziness, sedation, blurred vision, GI upset, rash	Hyponatremia in 2.5% of pts; derivative of carbamazepine that tends to be better tolerated and have less hepatic enzyme induction (may still decrease effectiveness of oral contraceptives)
Lamotrigine (Lamictal)	100-400 mg	None	Headache, dizziness, GI upset, blurred vision, rash	Stevens-Johnson syndrome (requires slow dose titration to minimize risk)

BUN=blood urea nitrogen; Cr=creatinine; CBC=complete blood count; TSH=thyroid stimulating hormone; ECG=electrocardiogram; LFTs=liver function tests; VPA=valproic acid; CBZ=carbamazepine; GI=gastrointestinal; SIADH=syndrome of inappropriate antidiuretic hormone

1. Olanzapine, risperidone, quetiapine, ziprasidone, and aripiprazole also have indications as mood stabilizers and are discussed in Table 3.

Table 3. Key Features of Antipsychotics

Medication	Usual Daily Dosing Range (mg)	Proposed Mechanism of Action	Side Effects	Other Key Features or Adverse Effects
Typical Antipsychotics[1] *Low Potency* Chlorpromazine (Thorazine) Thioridazine (Mellaril) *Mid Potency* Loxapine (Loxitane) *High Potency* Haloperidol (Haldol) Fluphenazine (Prolixin)	 300-600 300-600 45-90 5-15 5-15	Dopamine D_2 antagonism	Low potency: sedation, anticholinergic effects[2], orthostatic hypotension, weight gain, rarely agranulocytosis, lowered seizure threshold High potency: EPS Thioridazine: retrograde ejaculation, retinal pigmentation (doses > 800 mg/day)	NMS; TD (cumulative incidence of 5% per year of exposure among young adults and one year prevalence of 30% in elderly); hyperprolactinemia; torsade de pointes (thioridazine, chlorpromazine, rarely haloperidol)
Clozapine (Clozaril)	300-500	Weak D_2 antagonism + 5-HT_2 antagonism	Sedation, orthostatic hypotension, weight gain, lowered seizure threshold (dose-dependent), anticholinergic effects[2], hypersalivation, little to no risk of EPS	Agranulocytosis (1% of pts); requires weekly CBC for 6 mo, then biweekly CBC; treatment-emergent diabetes and hyperlipidemia
Risperidone (Risperdal)	3-6	D_2 antagonism + 5-HT_2 antagonism	Insomnia, hypotension, agitation, headache, EPS	Hyperprolactinemia; NMS; TD (less than typicals)

Medication	Usual Daily Dosing Range (mg)	Proposed Mechanism of Action	Side Effects	Other Key Features or Adverse Effects
Olanzapine (Zyprexa)	7.5-20	D_2 antagonism + 5-HT_2 antagonism	Sedation, weight gain, some EPS	Treatment-emergent diabetes and hyperlipidemia; NMS; TD (less than typicals)
Quetiapine (Seroquel)	400-800	D_2 antagonism + 5-HT_2 antagonism	Sedation, orthostatic hypotension, some weight gain, little EPS	Cataracts in beagle studies; TD (less than typicals); NMS
Ziprasidone (Geodon)	120-160	D_2 antagonism + 5-HT_2 antagonism	Headache, GI upset, sedation, EPS, little weight gain	Prolonged QTc greater than other atypicals; NMS; TD (less than typicals)
Aripiprazole (Abilify)	10-30	Partial agonist at D_2 + 5-HT_{1A} + antagonist at 5-HT_2	GI upset, headache, anxiety, sleep disturbance, EPS, little weight gain	Likely NMS; likely TD

D_2=dopamine type 2 receptor; 5-HT_2=serotonin type 2 receptor; 5-HT_{1A}=serotonin type 1A receptor; EPS=extrapyramidal symptoms; NMS=neuroleptic malignant syndrome; TD= tardive dyskinesia; GI=gastrointestinal; CBC=complete blood count

1. Representative typical antipsychotics are discussed here; this is an incomplete listing.
2. Anticholinergic side effects include dry mouth, blurred vision, constipation, urinary retention, tachycardia, and confusion.

Table 4. Key Features of Anxiolytics[1]

Medication	Dosing	Proposed Mechanism of Action	Side Effects	Other Key Features or Adverse Effects
Benzodiazepines Alprazolam (Xanax) Chlordiazepoxide (Librium) Clonazepam (Klonopin) Diazepam (Valium) Lorazepam (Ativan) Oxazepam (Serax) Temazepam (Restoril)	Dose Equivalents 0.5 10 0.25 5 1 15 5	Enhance the activity of the $GABA_A$ receptor by binding to the benzodiazepine receptor site to facilitate endogenous GABA in inhibiting neuronal excitability (effects are limited by the amount of endogenous GABA)	Sedation, dizziness, ataxia, impaired cognitive and motor performance	Most dangerous in combination with alcohol or barbiturates with marked drowsiness, disinhibition, respiratory depression; paradoxical agitation (esp in those with brain damage); possible increased risk of cleft palate in infants exposed *in utero*; prolonged use results in tolerance, dependence, and withdrawal effects; lorazepam, oxazepam, and temazepam (LOT) are not dependent on hepatic metabolism and are preferred in patients with hepatic disease
Buspirone (Buspar)	30-60mg per day	Partial agonist at $5\text{-}HT_{1A}$	Headache, nausea, nervousness, insomnia, dizziness	No cross-tolerance with benzodiazepines; non-addictive

$GABA_A$ =gamma-aminobutyric acid type A receptor; $5\text{-}HT_{1A}$ = serotonin type 1A receptor

1. All medications listed in Table1. Key Features of Antidepressants, except Bupropion, also have indications and/or efficacy as anxiolytics (usually requiring titration to the upper dosing range).

Appendix E
Psychiatric Emergencies

Delirium

Delirium is a medical diagnosis that is frequently made by a psychiatrist, who may be consulted for management of behavioral problems often exhibited by the delirious patient. In fact, delirium is the most common psychiatric syndrome encountered in general medical hospitals, affecting more than two million patients per year. Delirium must be diagnosed expeditiously, as this diagnosis signifies impending death in approximately 25% of cases. Mortality rates are 10-65% higher in delirious patients when compared to controls. Most physicians will be faced with diagnosing and treating patients with delirium so use your psychiatry rotation as an opportunity to learn more about this important syndrome.

Clinical Characteristics

- Disturbance of consciousness
  - Inattentiveness
  - Hyperalertness or hypoalertness
- Change in cognition
  - Impaired memory (recall and short term)
  - Disorientation
  - Hallucinations (especially visual)
- Waxing and waning course
- Acute or subacute onset
- Different motoric subtypes
  - Hyperactive
  - Hypoactive
  - Mixed

Differential Diagnosis of Delirium

Infectious

Withdrawal

Acute metabolic

Trauma

CNS pathology

Hypoxia

Deficiencies

Endocrinopathies

Acute vascular

Toxins, drugs, medications

Heavy metals

Treatment of delirium

Goals of Treatment
Identify and treat the underlying medical condition. Control inappropriate behaviors that endanger the patient and staff and interfere with the delivery of medical care.

Environmental Intervention
Continually reorient patient
Clocks, calendar, familiar objects
Private room with window
Adequate lighting
Eyeglasses, hearing aids

Supportive Care
Room near nursing station
Increased observation
Monitoring of VS, hydration, oxygenation
Discontinue all nonessential medications
Vigilance and constant follow up

Psychosocial Support
Family members present or supportive sitter
Reassure and educate patient and family

Pharmacologic Interventions
Haloperidol (PO, IM; IV not FDA approved)
Atypical Antipsychotics (PO, IM)
Avoid benzodiazepines, which may cause paradoxical agitation
Avoid anticholinergic agents, which may worsen confusion

Mechanical Restraints
For calm but confused patient performing dangerous maneuvers (pulling at IV, ET tube, etc)

Alcohol Withdrawal

Following the cessation or reduction of alcohol intake after prolonged and heavy use, patients may develop symptoms of alcohol withdrawal. In severe cases, alcohol withdrawal can be permanently disabling or fatal. This condition can be viewed as a spectrum including the following symptoms.

Early Withdrawal

- Onset 8-9 hours after last drink
- Autonomic hyperactivity
- Diaphoresis
- Tremor
- Insomnia
- Agitation
- Anxiety
- Nausea / vomiting
- Seizures
- Transient hallucinations or illusions (visual, tactile, auditory)

Alcohol Withdrawal Seizures

- Occur 24-48 hours after last drink
- May be related to hypoglycemia, hyponatremia, hypomagnesemia in chronic alcoholics

Delirium Tremens

- Onset 48-96 hours after last drink
- Tremor and increased psychomotor activity
- Vivid hallucinations
- Profound disorientation
- Increased autonomic activity and fever

Wernicke's Encephalopathy

- Confusion, ataxia, ophthalmoplegia, orthostasis

- Even partial thiamine supplementation may resolve eye signs, leaving AMS, ataxia and orthostasis

- Glucose poteniates symptoms, so thiamine needs to be administered first

- Untreated, it might progress to Korsakoff's Syndrome (persistent amnesia)

Nutritional Supplementation for Inpatient Detoxification

IM replacement immediately

- 1 amp MgSO4 (adjust for pts with, or predisposed to, renal insufficiency)
- Thiamine 100mg, folic acid 1mg, MVI

IV replacement to prevent delirium and seizures

- 3 liters of 5%D / 0.45saline at 200-300 cc/hr
- To each liter, add 1 amp of MVI, 6-8cc of MgSO4 (3-4mg of Mg),1 amp of trace minerals, 5mg folic acid, 200mg thiamine, KCl if vomiting

Daily oral nutritional supplementation

- Pyridoxine 50mg daily
- Thiamine 100mg daily
- MVI daily
- Folic acid 1mg daily
- Magnesium Oxide 400mg bid for 5 days (if hypomagnesemic)

Benzodiazepine Protocol for Inpatient Detoxification

May use chlordiazepoxide (Librium) or lorazepam
(Ativan); lorazepam is preferable in patients with liver
disease as it does not require hepatic metabolism.
Begin with lorazepam 2mg PO/IM or chlordiazepoxide
50mg PO/IM and repeat dose every 1-2 hours until the
patient is calm. On day 2 give the same total dose as day
1, divided into three doses. Taper the dose by 20% per
day over the next 5 days.

AgItation and Aggression

Patients on med/surg and psychiatric units or in the emergency room may become agitated for a variety of reasons. While determining the reason for the agitation or aggression is important, especially in cases such as delirium, the safety of the staff (including you) and the patient takes priority. The goal is to use the least restrictive intervention necessary, beginning with non-physical techniques first. If these techniques fail, physical intervention may become necessary. Oral medication should be offered to patients and emergency medication given if other interventions have failed. Before using medications, attempt to obtain or review vital signs, medical history, medication allergies and a brief visual examination of the patient (eyeball the patient).

Assess Cause of Aggression
Psychosis or mania
Delirium
Personality disorder
Manipulation for secondary gain

Constantly assess safety

Non-threatening Non-verbal Communication
Calm appearance
Appropriate eye contact
Relaxed body posture with open stance
Non-threatening hand gestures

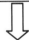

Verbal Intervention
Quiet, even tone of voice
Call the patient by name
Reassure and reorient the patient
Decrease the overall level of stimulation
Communicate an understanding of the patient's feelings
Present the natural consequences of the patient's threatening actions
Offer a problem-solving approach (How can I help you?)
Distract the patient away from the situation at hand
Use small talk to establish rapport
Offer food or drink
Offer medication

Physical Intervention
Include any staff member who has a good rapport with the patient
A "show of force" may be all that is required to deter the patient
Utilize all staff available, including security agents
Start with gentle physical redirection, escorting of the patient
Physical restraint may be required
Restraints should be discontinued as soon as possible

Pharmacological Intervention
Haloperidol (PO, IM)
Atypical antipsychotics (PO, IM)
Avoid benzodiazepines, except in withdrawal

Suicide

Suicidality is a common and serious problem in psychiatry as well as in general medical settings. In fact, the majority of people who commit suicide have seen their primary care doctor in the past six months and 70% saw their primary care physician in the month prior to suicide.

Populations at Increased Risk for Suicide

- Patients explicitly mentioning suicidal ideation
- Patients giving indirect clues to possible suicidal ideation:
     "No one would miss me if I were gone."
     "I would be better off dead."
     "This is probably the last time you'll see me."
- Recent losses
- Severe, chronic, or terminal medical illness
- High-risk psychiatric diagnoses: depression, bipolar disorder, schizophrenia, severe anxiety, substance abuse
- High-risk demographics: male sex, older age, single, widowed, divorced, unemployed, retired
- History of previous suicide attempts

Points to Remember When Asking About Suicide

- You will not plant the idea in the patient's mind. Use a gradual progression of questions…

     How much has this (illness, loss, problem) gotten you down?

     Do you sometimes feel like life is not worth living?

     Do you feel like giving up?

     Have you had thoughts about harming or killing yourself?

- Ask about details of suicide attempt or plan…

     How, When, Where? How determined is the patient?

     How feasible is the plan?

     Does the patient have access to lethal means?

Management of Suicidal Patients
Depends on severity of risk
Designed to protect the patient
Stable environment with supervision

- Family
- Voluntary hospitalization
- Involuntary hospitalization

Homicide

The homicidal patient is one who is threatening to kill a specific person(s). If this patient suffers from a mental illness that is influencing their homicidality, then measures must be taken to intervene so that the target is protected. Most often, this will involve detaining and hospitalizing the patient on an involuntary basis so that the mental illness may be treated. However, if a homicidal patient does not have a mental illness and does possess the capacity to make their own decisions, then the issue of homicidality becomes an issue requiring the attention of law enforcement authorities. One may inform the local police in this case. Issues of confidentiality and legal responsibility to warn threatened parties may come into conflict with one another. The duty of a physician to warn a third party of a patient's intent to harm varies depending upon the state, and you should investigate the details of this medical-legal issue in your own state.

Appendix F

Comprehensive Interview Template

This comprehensive interview template can be used to help you remember what areas to cover with each patient and can be photocopied to take with you into the evaluation. It will be especially useful to help you learn how to ask certain questions in the psychiatric review of symptoms and keep your interview conversational. You will probably not ask every patient every question contained in this template, but is will be a useful reference for you in approaching various patients.

CC

HPI

Psychiatric Review of Symptoms Screening Questions

Depression

Are you depressed?
Are the things that you normally enjoy still fun?
Any changes in sleep or appetite patterns?
Are you feeling guilty for things that others say are not your fault?

Mania

Have there been several days in a row when you didn't sleep and didn't need to?
Have your thoughts ever gone through your head so fast that you couldn't keep up with them?
Has anyone ever told you that you were talking so fast or about so many different things that they couldn't keep up with you?

Generalized Anxiety Disorder

Do you find yourself worrying about things that are out of your control?
Do people call you a "worrywart"?

Panic Disorder

Do you ever have extreme feelings of panic or fear that something terrible is happening?
Is this accompanied by shortness of breath, chest palpitations, dizziness, or other strange sensations in your body?

Obsessive-Compulsive Disorder

Do you have intrusive thoughts that disturb you and that you can't get out of your head?
Do you have to do certain rituals to get rid of the thoughts or to prevent something bad from happening?

PTSD

Have you experienced a traumatic event that you keep reliving in your thoughts or dreams?
How do you feel inside when you wake up?
Do you try to avoid things that remind you of this event?

Schizophrenia

Do you hear voices when you're alone or see things that other people don't?
Do you feel that someone is out to get you?
Do you get special messages from the television or radio?

Substance Abuse/Dependence

How often do you drink alcohol?
Do you drink until you are intoxicated or black out?
Have you ever had problems with withdrawal when you tried to stop or cut down on drinking?
Have you ever had seizures associated with drinking or withdrawing?
What drugs do you use?
Have you ever gotten into trouble with the law, an employer, or family member because of alcohol or drug use?

Past Psychiatric History

Past Medical History

Medications

Allergies

Family Psychiatric History

Social and Developmental History

Current Living Situation

Current Relationships/Support System

Family of Origin Relationships

Abuse History (physical, emotional, sexual)

Education/School Performance

Military Service

Legal History

Mental Status Exam

GENERAL APPEARANCE

☐ appears stated age ☐ older than stated age
☐ younger than stated age
☐ cachectic ☐ thin ☐ medium
☐ overweight ☐ obese ☐ morbidly obese

Dress: ☐ appropriate ☐ hospital dress
☐ street clothes ☐ sloppy ☐ odd_____

Eye Contact: ☐ good ☐ fair ☐ poor ☐ intense

Grooming: ☐ appropriate ☐ disheveled ☐ malodorous

Attitude: ☐ appropriate ☐ pleasant ☐ guarded
☐ suspicious ☐ paranoid
☐ angry ☐ anxious ☐ seductive ☐ hostile
☐ withdrawn ☐ _____

SENSORIUM

☐ alert ☐ drowsy ☐ stupor ☐ comatose
☐ oriented x 3 ☐ oriented only to _____

MOTOR

☐ no abnormalities ☐ retarded ☐ agitated
☐ abnormal movements _____

Gait: ☐ normal gait ☐ shuffling gait ☐ wide gait
☐ limping ☐ festinating

SPEECH

Rate: ☐ normal ☐ slow ☐ rapid ☐ pressured ☐ mute
☐ _____

Rhythm: ☐ normal ☐ monotonous ☐ stuttering
☐ broken ☐ _____

Volume: ☐ appropriate ☐ whispering ☐ soft
☐ loud ☐ _____

Articulation: ☐ appropriate ☐ mumbled ☐ slurred
☐ dysarthric ☐ _____

MOOD

Patient's words "_____"

COMPREHENSIVE INTERVIEW TEMPLATE

AFFECT
☐ appropriate ☐ full range ☐ constricted ☐ flat
☐ blunted ☐ labile
☐ euthymic ☐ happy ☐ expansive ☐ euphoric
☐ sad ☐ depressed ☐ dysphoric
☐ irritable ☐ anxious ☐ angry ☐ hostile

THOUGHT PROCESSES
☐ logical ☐ linear ☐ circumstantial ☐ tangential
☐ flight of ideas
☐ loose associations ☐ word salad ☐ concrete
☐ perseveration

THOUGHT CONTENT
☐ no SI ☐ life's not worth living ☐ + SI
☐ SI + plan _____
☐ no HI ☐ + HI ☐ HI + plan _____
☐ obsessions ☐ ruminations ☐ phobias
☐ ideas of reference ☐ thought insertion/withdrawal
☐ delusions ☐ paranoid ☐ grandiose ☐ somatic

PERCEPTUAL DISORDERS
☐ no abnormalities ☐ auditory hallucinations
☐ visual hallucinations ☐ illusions
☐ depersonalization ☐ derealization

INTELLECT
☐ average ☐ below average ☐ above average
☐ borderline retardation ☐ retardation

MEMORY
Immediate: ☐ intact ☐ impaired
Recent: ☐ intact ☐ impaired
Remote: ☐ intact ☐ impaired

CONCENTRATION
☐ intact ☐ distracted ☐ waxing and waning

INSIGHT
☐ good ☐ fair ☐ limited ☐ poor

JUDGMENT
☐ good ☐ fair ☐ limited ☐ poor

DSM-IV Diagnosis

Axis I:

Axis II:

Axis III:

Axis IV:

Axis V: GAF:

Treatment Plan

Appendix G

Global Assessment of Functioning

The Global Assessment of Functioning (GAF) is scored and placed on Axis V of the Multiaxial Assessment. To score the current GAF using the chart on the following pages, identify the most severe symptom(s) from your evaluation. Use the corresponding column on the scale to find the best description of the patient's symptom and assign a GAF score based on that symptom.

Example

A patient has frequent suicidal ideations but has not actually attempted suicide. She has thought of a plan but does not intend to act on it. Using the "Suicidal Thoughts or Actions" column, the best description of the patient's symptom would be "suicidal preoccupation with minimal danger," resulting in a GAF of 21-30.

This chart is adapted and reprinted with permission from the *Diagnostic and Statistical Manual of Mental Disorders, Fourth Edition, Text Revision*, Copyright 2000. American Psychiatric Association. Original adaptation courtesy of Joseph D. Hamilton, M.D.

GAF range	Suicidal Thoughts or Actions	Aggressive or Violent Behavior	Impaired Judgment
1-10	*Persistent danger* of *severely* hurting self or serious suicidal act with expectation of death	*Persistent danger* of *severely* hurting others (*e.g.*, recurrent violence)	Persistent danger of hurting self or others by impaired judgment (*e.g.*, repeatedly wanders into traffic)
11-20	*Some danger* of hurting self (*e.g.*, suicide attempt without clear expectation of death)	*Some danger* of hurting others	*Some danger* of hurting self or others by impaired judgment (*e.g.*, manic excitement)
21-30	Suicidal *preoccupation*, with minimal or no imminent danger of hurting self	Other violence with serious consequences	Other serious impairment in judgment (e.g., acts grossly inappropriately)
31-40			
41-50	*Suicidal ideation*, with minimal or no imminent danger of hurting self		
51-60			
61-70			
71-80			
81-90			
91-100			

160

Impaired Communication	Delusions or Hallucinations	Nonpsychotic Symptoms	Social & Occupational Functioning
			Persistent inability to maintain minimal personal hygiene
Gross impairment in communication (*e.g.,* incoherent or mute)			*Occasional failure* to maintain minimal personal hygiene (*e.g.,* smears feces)
Serious impairment in communication (*e.g.,* sometimes incoherent)	Behavior considerably influenced by delusions or hallucinations		*Inability to function* in almost *all* areas (*e.g.,* stays in bed all day, no job, home, or friends)
Some impairment in communications (*e.g.,* speech at times illogical or irrelevant)	Delusions or hallucinations without considerable influence on behavior		*Major impairment* in *several* areas, (*e.g.,* depressed man avoids friends, neglects family, and is unable to keep a job)
		Serious symptoms (*e.g.,* severe obsessions or depressed mood)	*Serious impairment* in *one area*: social, occupational, school functioning (*e.g.,* no friends or unable to work)
Mild impairment in communication (*e.g.,* circumstantial speech)		*Moderate symptoms* (*e.g.,* occasional panic attacks or moderate depressed mood)	*Moderate difficulty* in *one area*: social, occupational, school functioning (*e.g.,* few friends or conflicts with peers)
		Some *mild symptoms* (*e.g.,* mild depressed mood or mild insomnia)	Some difficulty in *one area*: social, occupational, school functioning, but generally functioning pretty well with some meaningful relationships
		Transient symptoms: expectable reactions to psychosocial stressors (*e.g.,* difficulty concentrating after argument)	No more than *slight difficulty* in *one area*: social or occupational or school functioning (*e.g.,* temporarily falling behind in schoolwork)
		Minimal symptoms (*e.g.,* mild anxiety before an exam)	Good functioning in all areas with no more than everyday problems or concerns
		No symptoms	Superior functioning in all areas

161

Appendix H

Evaluation of Cognitive Functioning

Any patient with suspected cognitive deficits should be screened with the mini-mental status examination (MMSE). Though this is not an adequate evaluation of all cognitive processes, it does assess such processes as orientation, memory, attention, and language. The score should be corrected based upon the patient's age and education level.

Corrected Scoring on the MMSE for Age and Education

Educational level

Age	0-4 yrs	5-8 yrs	9-12 yrs	College
18-24	22	27	29	29
25-29	25	27	29	29
30-34	25	26	29	29
35-39	23	26	28	29
40-44	23	27	28	29
45-49	23	26	28	29
50-54	23	27	28	29
55-59	22	26	28	29
60-64	23	26	28	29
65-69	22	26	28	29
70-74	22	25	27	28
75-79	21	25	27	28
80-84	20	25	25	27
> 84	19	23	26	27

Corrected scoring table adapted from Crum RM, Anthony JC, Bassett SB, Folstein MF. Population-based norms for the Mini-Mental State Examination by age and educational level. JAMA. 1993 May 12;269(18):2386-91.

Mini-Mental Status Examination

Orientation (score 1 for each correct)
    Name this hospital or building.   _____

    What floor of the building are you on?   _____

    What city are you in now?   _____

    What county is this?   _____

    What state are you in?   _____

    What year is it?   _____

    What month is it?   _____

    What is the date today?   _____

    What is the day of the week?   _____

    What season of the year is it?   _____

Registration (score 1 for each object repeated)
    "I'm going to say three things and I want you to   _____
    repeat them after me: ____, ____, ____."

Attention and Calculation (max score = 5)
    Subtract 7 from 100 in serial fashion to 65;   _____
    alternatively, ask them to spell WORLD
    backwards (have them spell it forwards first to
    check spelling ability).

Recall (score 1 for each object recalled)
    Do you remember the three objects named   _____
    before?

Language
    Confrontation naming: watch, pen = 2   _____
    Repetition: "No ifs, ands, or buts" = 1   _____
    Comprehension: "Point to the ceiling, after you   _____
    touch your nose" = 3
    Read and perform the following command: _____
    "close your eyes" = 1
    Write any sentence = 1   _____

Construction
    Copy the design below = 1   _____

Total MMSE Score (maximum = 30)   _____

MMSE adapted from Folstein MF, Folstein S, McHugh PR. "Mini-mental state." A practical method for grading the cognitive state of patients for the clinician. J Psychiatr Res. 1975 Nov;12(3):189-98.

163

Clock Drawing

The MMSE does not adequately assess all areas of cognition, especially executive functioning. Hence, patients may score in the normal range on the MMSE, yet still have significant cognitive disturbances. The clock drawing better tests a number of cognitive functions, including executive functioning, located primarily in the frontal lobes. It assesses auditory and graphomotor language skills, memory representation of a clock and the mechanism for retrieving this information, visuoperceptual and visuomotor processing, visuoperception to guide the layout of the clock and hemiattention to both sides of the space, parallel cognitive processing to allow both the writing of numbers and maintenance of their correct spatial layout, memory of the specific time setting, and executive functions of planning, organization, correcting, and simultaneous processing to coordinate the multiple steps. In addition to the frontal lobes, drawing versus copying a clock can localize deficits in other regions of the brain as well. Having a patient draw a clock to command places maximal demand on memory and visual imagery located in the temporal region. Asking the patient to copy a clock that you have drawn places maximal demand on the perceptual functions of the right parietal region.

Directions for Testing

1. Ask the patient to draw the face of a clock and to leave enough room to put in all of the numbers.

2. Ask the patient to draw in the hands of the clock, showing the time, "10 past 11."

3. You may also ask the patient to copy a clock you have drawn.

Scoring

There are two methods for scoring these drawings, and we include the method described by Sunderland and colleagues here, as we find it more useful. You should also describe the clock drawing, including what the patient did correctly and incorrectly, as the scoring system may not be meaningful to everyone who reads the chart.

The Sunderland Method

Normal Example

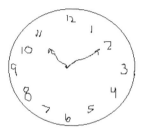

Score = 10

Abnormal Example

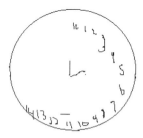

Score = 5

Score	Criterion

10 - 6   **Drawing of clock face is generally intact.**

10   Hands are in the correct position.

9   Slight errors in placement of the hands.

8   Moderate errors in placement of the hands.

7   Significant errors in placement of the hands.

6   Inappropriate use of hands (i.e., no hands present, circling of number.)

5 - 1   **Drawing of clock face is not intact.**

5   Crowding of numbers at one end of the clock or reversal of numbers. Hands may still be present in some fashion.

4   Numbers may be missing or placed outside the clock face. Clock face lacks integrity.

3   Numbers have no relation to the circle.

Hands are not present.

2   Patient shows some understanding of directions with his or her attempt to draw the clock, but draws only a vague representation of a clock.

1   No attempt or interpretable results.

101 Biggest Mistakes 3rd Year Medical Students Make and How to Avoid Them

ISBN # 0-9725561-0-9

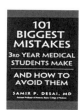

Compiled from discussions with hundreds of attending physicians, residents, and students, the *101 Biggest Mistakes 3rd Year Medical Students Make And How To Avoid Them* discusses the major mistakes that students make during this very important year. Avoiding these pitfalls is the key to third year success. This book will empower you, placing you in a position to have a successful experience, no matter what rotation or clerkship you are on. Once you are aware of these mistakes, you can do everything in your power to avoid them, thereby becoming the savvy student that is poised for clerkship success. Read what others have had to say:

"As someone who just matched into dermatology, I can tell you that residency program directors look closely at clerkship grades, especially for the more competitive residencies. *101 Biggest Mistakes 3rd Year Medical Students Make And How To Avoid Them* is a book that will help you get great clerkship grades."

Review posted by Yang Xia on www.amazon.com.

The Residency Match: 101 Biggest Mistakes And How To Avoid Them

ISBN # 0-9725561-1-7

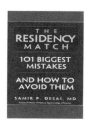

Are there any steps you can take to maximize your chances of matching with the residency program of your choice? One of the keys is to become familiar with the major mistakes that students make during the residency application process. These are mistakes that are well known to residency program directors but are not familiar to many applicants. In *The Residency Match: 101 Biggest Mistakes And How To Avoid Them*, we not only show you these mistakes but also help you avoid them, placing you in a position for match success. Read what others have had to say:

"The fourth year of medical school can be a stressful, demanding time. This book cuts down on the amount of necessary reading that you must do in order to match well. It has tips about subjects I had not thought about (for example, you should have a case ready to present your interviewer), as well as questions you will be asked in interviews and questions you should ask the interviewer. Overall, this is an easy to read book that I would definitely recommend because it contains all the essentials to matching in your ideal residency spot."

Review posted by Jonathan Welch on www.amazon.com

Pediatrics Clerkship: 101 Biggest Mistakes And How To Avoid Them
ISBN # 0-9725561-4-1

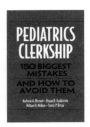

The Pediatrics Clerkship is different in many respects from every other core clerkship, and many students are uncertain of how to success-fully navigate the transition from adult care to the care of children. Students are often unsure of how to take a pediatric history, perform a physical examination, produce a comprehen-sive pediatric write-up, see patients in the out-patient setting, and take care of patients in the nursery. This book will ease the transition by introducing you to the all-too-common mistakes that are made during the clerk-ship. With this knowledge in hand, you will become a more productive team member at an earlier point in the rotation, ready to fully focus on learning the fundamentals of pediatric medicine.

Internal Medicine Clerkship: 150 Biggest Mistakes And How To Avoid Them

ISBN # 0-9725561-2-5

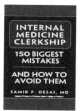

Did you know that most medical students begin doing their best work at the end of the Internal Medicine clerkship? Wouldn't it be great if there were a book available that could speed up the learning curve so that students were performing at a high level right from the get-go? Now with the *Internal Medicine Clerkship: 150 Biggest Mistakes And How To Avoid Them*, there's absolutely no reason to save your best for last. Read what others have had to say:

"I read the book cover to cover prior to starting the rotation, and it helped me get off to a great start. I feel the book had a great influence on both my performance as a clinical student and my evaluation by my teammates. Overall, an extremely helpful and eye opening text. I attribute much of my success to the wisdom I gathered from this book."

—Brian Broaddus, after completing his Internal Medicine clerkship at the Baylor College of Medicine

Surgery Clerkship: 150 Biggest Mistakes And How To Avoid Them

ISBN # 0-9725561-3-3

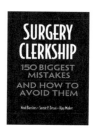

At most medical schools, the surgery clerkship is considered to be the most difficult rotation. Days start early, end late, and, from start to finish, the work is intense and demanding, often leading to physical and mental exhaustion. Of course, this can negatively impact your learning, enjoyment, and performance during the clerkship. To prevent this from happening, turn to the *Surgery Clerkship: 150 Biggest Mistakes and How To Avoid Them*, a resource that will help you overcome the challenges that await you. Lessen your anxiety, alleviate your fears, and position yourself for success by turning to the only book that will help you with every facet of the rotation, including not only your day to day patient care responsibilities but also your preparation for the oral and NBME clerkship exams.

MD2B Titles

101 Biggest Mistakes 3rd Year Medical Students Make And How To Avoid Them

The Residency Match: 101 Biggest Mistakes And How To Avoid Them

Internal Medicine Clerkship: 150 Biggest Mistakes And How To Avoid Them

Surgery Clerkship: 150 Biggest Mistakes And How To Avoid Them

Pediatrics Clerkship: 101 Biggest Mistakes And How To Avoid Them

Psychiatry Clerkship: 150 Biggest Mistakes And How To Avoid Them

View sample chapters of these books at www.md2b.net

About www.md2b.net

Our website, www.md2b.net, is committed to helping today's medical student become tomorrow's doctor. The site is dedicated to providing students with the tools needed to tackle the challenges of medical school. The website provides the following information:

      Survival Guides for 3rd Year Clerkships

      Success tips (tips of the week)

      Introduction to the residency match

      Residency Match tips

                AND MUCH MORE!